REVERSING
DIABETES

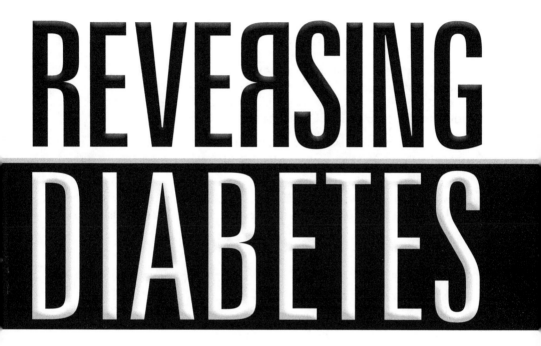

REVERSING DIABETES

DON COLBERT, MD

SILOAM

Most CHARISMA HOUSE BOOK GROUP products are available at special quantity discounts for bulk purchase for sales promotions, premiums, fund-raising, and educational needs. For details, write Charisma House Book Group, 600 Rinehart Road, Lake Mary, Florida 32746, or telephone (407) 333-0600.

REVERSING DIABETES by Don Colbert, MD
Published by Siloam
Charisma Media/Charisma House Book Group
600 Rinehart Road
Lake Mary, Florida 32746
www.charismahouse.com

Unless otherwise noted, all Scripture quotations are from the New King James Version of the Bible. Copyright © 1979, 1980, 1982 by Thomas Nelson, Inc., publishers. Used by permission.

Scripture quotations marked NLT are from the New Living Translation of the Bible, copyright © 1996, 2004. Used by permission of Tyndale House Publishers, Inc., Wheaton, IL 60189. All rights reserved.

Cover design by Justin Evans
Design Director: Bill Johnson

Visit the author's website at www.drcolbert.com.

Library of Congress Cataloging-in-Publication Data

Colbert, Don.
  Reversing diabetes / Don Colbert.
      p. cm.
  Includes bibliographical references and index.
    ISBN 978-1-61638-598-9 (trade paper) -- ISBN 978-1-61638-705-1 (ebook)
  1. Diabetes--Alternative treatment. 2. Diabetes--Diet therapy 3.
Diabetes--Prevention. 4. Naturopathy. I. Title.
  RC661.A47C65 2012
  616.4'62--dc23

                              2011047098

Portions of this book were previously published as *Dr. Colbert's "I Can Do This" Diet* by Siloam, ISBN 978-1-61638-267-4, copyright © 2010, and *The New Bible Cure for Diabetes* by Siloam, ISBN 978-1-59979-759-5, copyright © 2009.

CONTENTS

Section III: It All Begins With "Waist Management"

Section IV: Reversing Type 2 Diabetes Through Diet

Section V: Other Important Steps in Reversing Type 2 Diabetes

TYPE 2 DIABETES *CAN* BE REVERSED!

God's desire is for you to feel better and to live longer—and He will help you reach that goal! By picking up this book, you have taken a major step toward renewed energy and health. This will enable you to fight back against diabetes, which is afflicting millions of people at an ever-younger age. If you are prediabetic, this book is preventive, helping you avoid type 2 diabetes. If you have type 1 diabetes, the advice in this book can help you manage your glucose levels and ward off the long-term complications associated with the disease. However, you will require insulin injections daily. And if you have type 2 diabetes, this book can help you restore your health and many times reverse the disease.

You may be confronting the greatest physical challenge of your life. But with faith in God, good nutrition, and cutting-edge natural remedies, reversing diabetes can represent a great victory in your life! God revealed His divine will for each of us through the apostle John, who wrote, "Beloved, I pray that you may prosper in all things and be in health, just as your soul prospers" (3 John 2).

Nearly two thousand years later, nearly 26 million American adults suffer from a disease called diabetes—and a fourth of them don't even know they have it![1] Researchers at the Centers for Disease Control and Prevention (CDC) recently made the stunning revelation that during the 2005–2008 time period, 35 percent of US adults age twenty or older had prediabetes, including 50 percent of those over sixty-five. Applying those percentages to the entire population yield an estimated 79 million Americans with prediabetes. Add diabetics and prediabetics together, and approximately one-third of our population, or 103 million, have prediabetes or diabetes. In addition, some 215,000 people under age twenty have type 1 or type 2 diabetes, the latter formerly considered an adult-onset problem. The CDC had already projected that without changes in diet and exercise, one in three children born in the United States in the year 2000 are likely to develop type 2 diabetes at some point during their lives.[2]

Why are we seeing such dramatic increases? It can be traced directly to the nation's obesity epidemic: two-thirds of American adults are overweight or obese, and 30 percent of children age eleven or younger are overweight.[3] This ought to alarm everyone, particularly everyone who professes Jesus as Savior and Lord. Surely we are missing God's best. Why? The conventional answer: many physicians are looking for the next new-and-improved medication. I suggest that is not a solution. We need to get to the *root* of the problem, which is our diet, lifestyle, and waistline. Without addressing this reality, the alarming toll from diabetes will only get worse.

Fast food, junk food, convenience foods, sodas, sweetened coffee drinks, sugar-laden juices, smoothies, "supersize" portions, and skipping meals all contribute to the problem. The standard American diet is full of empty carbohydrates, sugars, fats, excessive proteins, and calories, and it is low in nutrient content. This diet literally causes us to lose nutrients such as chromium, which is crucial in regulating glucose levels in our blood. To put it simply: people suffering from diabetes have high sugar levels in their blood.

Combined with our poor diet is a lack of physical activity. Too many children no longer play sports and participate in outdoor activities. Instead they get entranced by video games, smartphones, text messages, social networking, online media, TV shows, and movies. Combined with their favorite fast food, reducing exercise to a flick of the finger spells ever-increasing weight gain.

Also, the excessive stress that most adults and many children labor under increases cortisol levels. As a result, many are developing toxic belly fat, thereby increasing their risk for incurring diabetes. Long-term stress eventually depletes stress hormones as well as neurotransmitters. This often helps unleash ravenous appetites, plus addictions to sugar and carbohydrates. It's like a nightmarish vortex, each bad habit working to ensnare sufferers in a downward spiral to poor health and disease.

Type 2 Diabetes Is a "Choice" Disease

Galatians 6:7–8 says, "Do not be deceived, God is not mocked; for whatever a man sows, that he will also reap. For he who sows to his flesh will of the flesh reap corruption, but he who sows to the Spirit will of the Spirit reap everlasting life." Most Americans are unknowingly sowing seeds for a harvest of obesity, diabetes, and a host of other diseases by their choices of food and lifestyle habits.

The onset of type 1 diabetes is beyond anyone's control. However, I often say that prediabetes and type 2 diabetes are "choice" diseases. In other words, you *catch* a cold or the flu, but because of wrong choices you *develop* obesity, prediabetes, and type 2 diabetes.

Hosea 4:6 says, "My people are destroyed for lack of knowledge." My previous books *The Seven Pillars of Health* and *Dr. Colbert's "I Can Do This" Diet* provide a foundation for changing dietary patterns, improving lifestyle habits, and losing weight—especially the toxic belly fat closely related to diabetes. I encourage you to read *The Seven Pillars of Health*. The principles it contains are a foundation for healthy living that will affect all areas of your life. It sets the stage for everything you will ever read in any other book I've published, including this one.

In this book, *Reversing Diabetes*, you will learn about natural ways to avoid and usually reverse diabetes through diet, supplements, and exercise if you change dietary and lifestyle habits in time. You will also learn about the different types of diabetes, how this disease develops, and the complications of diabetes as it damages—and may eventually destroy—the kidneys, leading to dialysis. It also damages blood vessels and may lead to blindness, impotence, heart attack, stroke, and poor circulation in the extremities. It can damage nerves, leading to burning pains in the feet (as if someone were constantly burning you with cigarettes), numbness in the feet, foot and leg ulcers, infections, and possibly eventual amputation.

Is this helping you get the picture? Habitual consumption of soft drinks, candy bars, pie or cake, or large helpings of white rice, potatoes, and white bread will help you sign on the dotted line for prediabetes and diabetes.

Over the years I have seen patients stressed out over signing a contract without reading the small print. A few years ago a patient came in burning with anger because after moving out of his apartment, he discovered that he owed the owners an extra $1,000. He said that he never had to pay after leaving other apartment complexes. The manager replied, "Read your contract." When he did, my patient saw the extra-fine print that stipulated when an occupant left his apartment, he would have to pay $1,000.

In the same way millions of Americans are unknowingly signing up for diabetes, accompanied by all of the complications associated with this disease. Wake up. Take action while there is still time to reverse the curse of prediabetes and diabetes.

You may be wondering if there is any hope. The answer is yes! Your body is fearfully and wonderfully made. Regardless of which type of diabetes you or a loved one may have, God can heal either condition without difficulty. I have known people who were healed of diabetes by God's miracle-working power. I have witnessed others whose lives have dramatically improved through healthy lifestyle choices and natural treatments. Realize that God generally won't do what you can do yourself. After all, only you can choose to eat healthy foods, exercise, lose weight, and take supplements.

Since publication of *The Bible Cure for Diabetes* in 1999, many new things about diabetes came to light; many terms used to identify this illness changed. A decade later, I wrote *The New Bible Cure for Diabetes* with revised and updated information. Material from that book has been combined with parts of *Dr. Colbert's "I Can Do This" Diet* and other relevant, updated material. I wanted to offer medical information and practical insights on ways to reduce your waistline, control your weight, and take other commonsense steps to prevent, manage, and yes, even *reverse* diabetes.

There is much you can do to prevent or defeat diabetes. Now is the time to run to the battle with fresh confidence, renewed determination, and the wonderful knowledge that God is real, alive, and more powerful than any sickness or disease. It is my prayer that my suggestions and guidelines will help improve your health, nutritional habits, and fitness practices. This combination will bring wholeness to your life. I pray that they will deepen your fellowship with God and strengthen your ability to worship and serve Him.

—Don Colbert, MD

Section 1

UNDERSTANDING YOUR ENEMY

Chapter 1

THE DIABETES EPIDEMIC

When New York filmmaker Morgan Spurlock set out to draw a line between the rise of obesity in America and fast-food giant McDonald's, he never dreamed that his *Super Size Me* documentary would be nominated for an Academy Award, earn more than $20 million worldwide on a $65,000 production budget, and turn the film's title into a watchword for health activists around the globe. In short, he became McDonald's worst nightmare, one accentuated by the release of his ensuing memoir, *Don't Eat This Book.*

Spurlock's unexpected entry into international consciousness originated with a personal experiment, using himself as the guinea pig. For one month he ate nothing but McDonald's food for all three meals, in the process sampling every item on the Golden Arches' menu. Whenever cashiers asked if he wanted his meal supersized, he accepted.

When I first heard of his hypothesis, I found it a bit exaggerated. That is, until I realized that his experiment represented untold millions who get the majority of their daily sustenance from fast food. Spurlock turned himself into a physical representation of these silent masses, consuming an average of 5,000 calories a day. As a result, he gained almost 25 pounds, increased his body mass index by 13 percent, raised his cholesterol to 230, and accumulated fat in his liver. He turned his experiment into a statement heard around the world.[1]

Years later, I sometimes wonder if many Americans were paying attention. After reports in recent years of a stabilization in obesity rates, a report released by the Centers for Disease Control and Prevention (CDC) in the summer of 2011 showed they had inched up 1.1 percent between 2007 and 2009, leaving them at staggering levels of 33.8 percent.[2] The proportion of obese Americans is at astounding levels, about one-third or 33.8 percent.[3] Obesity currently kills an estimated four hundred thousand Americans a year and is the second-leading cause of preventable deaths in this nation.[4] The number one avoidable killer? Cigarette smoking (and a recent report shows it dropped 40 percent between 1965 and 2007).[5] That means losing weight ranks up there with quitting smoking as the most crucial lifestyle change you could ever make. Because of the lowered smoking trend, I predict that obesity will soon pass smoking as the number one avoidable killer of Americans.

Unfortunately, many doctors, nutritionists, and dietitians seem to either miss this fact or conveniently ignore it. They love to offer topical "Band-Aids" that alleviate patients' symptoms yet fail to tackle the root issues or consider the long-term ramifications of neglecting their patients' weight. A CDC report in 2007 found that about a third of obese adults had never been told by a doctor or health-care provider that they were obese.[6] Not only is this unbelievable, but obesity is also a key link to another serious, life-threatening issue: diabetes.

Diabetes kills more people than AIDS and breast cancer combined. It reportedly ranks as the seventh leading cause of death by disease among adults in America.[7] The sad reality is that it may rank much higher because research shows that diabetes is underreported, only being listed on 10 to 15 percent of death certificates as an underlying cause of death.[8]

The World Health Organization (WHO) estimates that by 2030, the worldwide number of individuals with diabetes will double. That means we could see the number of people suffering from diabetes reach 360 million within the next two decades.[9] And, within the United States, type 2 diabetes is increasing at an alarming rate. Not only do approximately one in every ten Americans age twenty and older have diabetes,[10] the rate of children being diagnosed with type 2 diabetes is growing at an alarming rate.

Such alarming information speaks for itself. Indeed, it is screaming while far too many practitioners turn the other way. With our nation facing the biggest health-care crisis in its history, each of us must realize that the answer won't come from doctors, clinics, or the US government. Instead, each person must take responsibility for his or her health. Because obesity and overweight conditions are at the root of so many health conditions, particularly diabetes, it makes sense to start by reducing to a healthy weight and a healthy waistline.

Defining the Problem

Before I delve into what has so many people visiting the plus-size department and developing diabetes along the way, I need to clarify the terms "overweight" and "obese." Many people have a general sense as to how these words are different, yet in recent years the delineation has become clearer. Various health organizations, including the CDC and the National Institutes of Health (NIH), now officially define them using the body mass index (BMI), which evaluates a person's weight relative to height. Most of these organizations define an overweight adult as having a BMI between 25 and 29.9, while an obese adult is anyone with a BMI of 30 or higher.[11]

Only a small portion of individuals who are overweight or obese according to their BMI have a normal or low body fat percentage. For example, professional athletes often have a high-muscle, low-body-fat makeup that causes them to weigh more than the average person, yet they are not truly obese (excluding some football linemen and sumo wrestlers). However, most people who come to me seeking help are not just overweight but technically obese—meaning males with body fat greater than 25 percent and females over 33 percent.[12] Throughout this book when I discuss having a high BMI, I will be referring to obese people, not those few muscular types with a high BMI but normal or low body fat.

Calories Cost

Researchers have discovered that for every extra 100 calories a person eats each day, the additional expenses—such as health care for future health problems caused by being obese—range from forty-eight cents to two dollars. Each time you supersize your meal for "only" thirty-five cents more, it can actually end up costing you between eighty-two cents and six dollars and sixty-four cents in health-care bills.

When everything is considered, obesity comes with a fat price tag (pun intended), with people considered obese paying $1,429 more (42 percent) in health-care costs than normal weight individuals. Expenses for each obese senior run Medicare $1,723 more than for normal weight beneficiaries, and private insurers $1,140 more.[13] Several years ago Seattle University management professor William L. Weis calculated the total annual revenue from the "obesity industry"—which includes fast-food restaurants, obesity-related medical treatments, and diet books—at more than $315 billion. That amounted to nearly 3 percent of the United States' economy![14]

According to author Michael Pollan, diabetes subtracts roughly twelve years from one's life, while someone living with the condition incurs annual medical costs of $13,000, compared to $2,500 for a person without diabetes. And although an estimated 80 percent of cases of type 2 diabetes are preventable with proper diet and exercise, he says the smart money is on the creation of a vast new industry: "Apparently it is easier, or at least a lot more profitable, to change a disease of civilization into a lifestyle than it is to change the way that civilization eats."[15]

Our nation's habit of ignoring solutions to focus on profits would almost be amusing if it wasn't so serious. And, as shocking as all this sounds, no dollar amount can do justice to the real damage being done. Being over-weight or obese increases your risk of developing thirty-five major dis-eases, particularly type 2 diabetes. And among others: heart disease, stroke, arthritis, hypertension, Alzheimer's disease, infertility, erectile dysfunction, and gallbladder disease. Plus more than a dozen forms of cancer. If you are an obese woman, you have a significantly higher risk of postmenopausal breast cancer—one and a half times more than a woman with an average healthy weight. You also increase your chances of developing uterine cancer because of your weight. For pregnant mothers, the risk of delivering a baby with a serious birth defect is doubled if you are overweight and quadrupled if you are obese.[16]

Besides obesity's physical implications, it carries a social and psycho-logical impact. Obese individuals generally contend with more rejection and prejudice. Often they are overlooked for promotions or not even hired because of physical appearance. Most obese people struggle daily with issues of self-worth and self-image. They feel unattractive and unappreci-ated and are at an increased risk of depression. Many of us have watched the humiliation an obese person experiences trying to squeeze into an air-plane, stadium, or automobile seat that is too small. Maybe you have been that person. If so, you know how obesity can affect the way others treat you and how you treat yourself.

Globesity Is the Culprit

Tragically, millions of others outside the United States struggle with the same issues. The World Health Organization calls obesity a worldwide epi-demic. Obesity and its expanding list of health consequences (led by dia-betes) is overtaking infection and malnutrition as the main cause of death and disability in many third-world nations. This "globesity," as Morgan Spurlock aptly points out in his documentary, has a major cause: the spread of fast food.

In his award-winning book *Fast Food Nation*, author Eric Schlosser chronicled how Americans spent about $6 billion on fast food in 1970, but by the turn of the century shelled out more than $110 billion. Because cor-porate America is a global trendsetter, other countries have followed suit. Between 1984 and 1993, the number of fast-food restaurants in Great Britain doubled. So did adults' obesity rate. Fast-forward fifteen years, and the British were eating more fast food than any other nation in Western Europe.

Meanwhile the proportion of overweight teens in China has roughly tri-pled in the past decade. In Japan, the obesity rate among children doubled during the 1980s, which correlated with a 200 percent increase in fast-food sales. This generation of Japanese has gone on to become the first in that traditionally slender Asian nation's history—thanks to its past proclivity for vegetables, rice, and fish—to be known for its bulging waistlines. By the year 2000, approximately one-third of all Japanese men in their thirties were overweight.[17] By adopting our fast-food habits, the entire world is beginning to look more like Americans. I fear that its diabetes rates will soon follow.

A Child Shall Lead Them

How has an entire generation of hefty eaters changed the face of the world? By starting young. Once again this unflattering trend originated in America. As I mentioned in the introduction, according to a 2011 CDC report, nearly twenty-six million people have diabetes, or 8.3 percent of the US population. In an earlier report, the CDC projected that one out of three children who were born in the United States in the year 2000 will develop type 2 diabetes at some point in their life.[19]

As a result of childhood obesity, the numbers of children with type 2 diabetes is rapidly rising across the country. And because of the connection of obesity to hypertension, high cholesterol, and heart disease, experts are predicting a dramatic rise in heart disease as our children become adults. The CDC reports that overweight teens stand a 70 percent chance of becoming overweight adults, which increases to 80 percent if at least one parent is obese or overweight. Because of that, heart disease and type 2 diabetes are expected to begin at a much earlier age among those who fail to beat the odds.[20] Today's generation of children is not expected to live as long as their parents, and they will be more likely to suffer from disease and illness at an earlier age.

So if you don't want to lose weight for yourself, at least do it for your children. Children follow by example by mirroring their parents' behavior. Don't tell them to lose weight if you aren't doing it yourself. I'm sure most of you are good parents and love your children. Yet you have to ask yourself: Do I love them enough to teach them what foods to eat and what foods to

TRENDS IN CHILDHOOD OBESITY

Research shows that childhood obesity tripled over the past thirty years. Obesity among children ages six to eleven tripled from 1980 to 2008, jumping from 6.5 percent to 19.6 percent. The rate rose even faster for those twelve to nineteen, increasing from 5 percent to 18.1 percent. Seventy percent of obese youth have at least one risk for cardiovascular disease. They are also likely to become obese adults, increasing their risk of associated health problems—diabetes among them.[18]

avoid? Do I love them enough to keep junk food out of the house while making healthy food available? Do I love them enough to engage in physical activity and lead by example?

If you answered yes to those questions, it is important that you take action for your children's sake. And your own. Not a "crash diet, quick fix" method but permanent lifestyle changes. I am thrilled that you have picked up this book because I believe you hold the key to truly changing your life and reversing diabetes, whether yours or the early signs appearing in your children. However, to be frank, this will not be an easy fight when it involves your children. They are growing up in a culture saturated with junk food that is void of nutrition and high in toxic fats, sugar, highly processed carbohydrates, and food additives and that is not only widely available but also heavily advertised.

To add to the challenge, they are surrounded by peers who consider consuming this junk natural and a normal part of childhood. For example, in 1978, the typical teen male in the United States drank 7 ounces of soda a day; today he drinks approximately three times that much. Meanwhile, he gets about a quarter of his daily servings of vegetables from french fries and potato chips.[25]

THE LINK TO ILLNESSES

- More than 90 percent of people who are newly diagnosed with type 2 diabetes are overweight or obese.[21]
- Obesity increases your risk of developing the following cancers: esophageal, thyroid, colon, kidney, prostate, endometrial, gallbladder, rectal, breast, pancreatic, leukemia, multiple myeloma, malignant melanoma, and non-Hodgkin's lymphoma.[22]
- Being overweight increases your risk of having GERD (acid reflux) symptoms by 50 percent; being obese doubles your chances.[23]
- Excess weight is also commonly known to cause sleep apnea and hypertension (high blood pressure). In fact, 75 percent of all cases hypertension in the United States is attributed to obesity.[24]

If you plan to take a stand against this garbage-in, garbage-out culture, expect opposition on every front. During the course of a year, the typical American child will watch more than thirty thousand TV commercials, many of them pitching fast food or junk food as delicious "must-eats." For years, fast-food franchises have enticed children into their restaurants with kids' meal toys, promotional giveaways, and elaborate playgrounds. This has worked perfectly for McDonald's: about 90 percent of American children between the ages of three and nine set foot in one each month.[26] When they can't visit the Golden Arches or another favored outlet, it comes to them.

Fast-food products—most brought in by franchisees—are sold in about 30 percent of public high school cafeterias and many elementary cafeterias.[27]

Because they spend billions of dollars on research and marketing, these fast-food establishments know exactly what they are doing and how to push your child's hot button. They understand the powerful impact certain foods can have on people at an early age. Have you ever thought about when you first started liking certain foods? Most people formed these preferences during the first few years of their

WORLD HUNGER

McDonald's feeds an astounding forty-seven million people a day worldwide. That is more than the entire populations of Canada and Cambodia combined![28]

lives. This is why comfort foods often do more than just fill the stomach. They evoke such memories as playgrounds, toys, backyard birthday bashes, Fourth of July parties, state fairs, and childhood friends. The aroma of onion rings, doughnuts, or grilled burgers can instantly trigger these memories. As adults, such smells often draw us without us recognizing their lure. Advertisers have keyed into this and learned to use the sight of food to stimulate fond childhood memories.

In the Genes or in the Water?

Every obese person has a story behind his or her excessive weight gain. Growing up, I often heard people say things like "she was born fat" or "he takes after his daddy."

There's some truth in both comments. When it comes to obesity, genetics count.

In 1988 the *New England Journal of Medicine* published a Danish study that observed 540 people adopted during infancy. The research found that adopted individuals had a much greater tendency to end up in the weight class of their biological parents rather than their adoptive parents.[29] Separate studies of twins raised apart also show that genetics has a strong influence on weight gain and becoming overweight.[30] Such studies reveal there is a significant genetic predisposition to gaining weight.

However, they still don't fully explain the epidemic of obesity seen in the United States the past thirty years. Although an individual may have a genetic predisposition to become obese, environment also plays a major role. I like the way author, speaker, and noted women's physician Pamela Peeke puts it: "Genetics may load the gun, but environment pulls the trigger."[31] Many patients I see come into my office thinking since they have inherited their "fat genes," there is nothing they can do. Yet, after a little investigation,

I usually find that they have inherited their parents' propensity for bad food choices, large portion sizes, and poor eating habits.

If you have been overweight since childhood, you probably have an increased number of fat cells. This means you will have a tendency to gain weight if you choose the wrong types of foods and large portions and fail to exercise. However, you should also realize that most people can override a genetic predisposition for obesity by making correct dietary and lifestyle choices. A parent's diabetes does not automatically condemn a child to the same disease, no matter how many people remark, "The apple doesn't fall far from the tree."

Unfortunately, many of us forget that to make these healthy choices, we need to place ourselves in a healthy environment. That is becoming more difficult than ever as families yield to hectic routines that feature grabbing breakfast on the way out the door, fast-food lunches, dining out for dinner, and sometimes skipping meals. Years of such habits are catching up to us. Starting at age twenty-five, the average American adult gains 1 to 3 pounds a year. That means a twenty-five-year-old, 120-pound female can expect to weigh anywhere between 150 and 210 pounds by the time she is fifty-five.

Is there any wonder we have an epidemic of heart disease, type 2 diabetes, hypertension, high cholesterol, arthritis, cancer, and other degenerative diseases? We have to put the brakes on this obesity epidemic—and a lifestyle approach to eating is the answer!

Eating With the Head, Not the Heart

The fact that obesity can stem from heredity, environment, and culture can feel discouraging, even overwhelming. How can one hope to overcome such powerful forces and reverse diabetes in the process? As tough as it may seem, there is cause for hope. I want to end this chapter on a positive note by reminding you of a simple truth. In fact, it is one of the primary reasons for this book.

It may sound impossible, but with education, practice, and discipline, your cultural tastes and dietary practices can gradually change. You can learn to choose similar foods that have not been highly processed and lower-fat alternatives. It is possible to discover—or rediscover—portion control and healthy cooking methods. What about fried

> **ENSALADA**
>
> Just because a taco salad features the word *salad* doesn't mean it's healthy. With the massive fried tortilla shell, beef, cheese, sour cream, and additional items (plus the nutritionally useless iceberg lettuce), most taco salads add up to about 900 calories and 55 grams of fat.

chicken, mashed potatoes and gravy, and chocolate cake? You can learn to enjoy the same foods, but with just a fraction of the fat, sugar, and calories.

When I wrote a book about the Mediterranean diet, *What Would Jesus Eat?*, I learned that most Middle Easterners eat differently than does the typical American. That sounds obvious, but what distinguishes the two isn't. I found that those who are used to a Mediterranean diet typically do not leave the dinner table stuffed as most Americans do. Generally, they eat anything they want—but in moderation. They enjoy their food at a leisurely pace, socializing while eating. They have the uncanny ability to enjoy just a few bites of such foods as wine, dark chocolate, and chocolate ice cream. Unlike most Americans, who scarf down a dessert as if they were inhaling it, those eating the Mediterranean way generally savor just a few bites.

The real pleasure in most foods is in the first few bites. If you remember nothing else in this book, remember this truth: you can break old, culturally based eating patterns. You do not have to follow a parent's poor food choices, and you can overcome your family's dietary cultural patterns. (I certainly did!) In the process you will discover the true joy of eating.

Chapter 2

TYPES OF DIABETES

The iPad and similar twenty-first-century notebooks are so prevalent today that some companies and organizations require that employees carry them to seminars and conferences. Watch televised election returns from the latest presidential or congressional races, and you will see the anchors and field reporters checking electronic updates, whether on an electronic notebook or smartphone. Small wonder that the assumption is that everyone in the modern era checks their apps and other devices to stay abreast of up-to-the-minute developments, even as young adults show signs that they are stressed out by the flood of gizmos they are expected to master. In the fall of 2010, an annual survey of college freshmen by UCLA showed their emotional health had fallen to its lowest levels in twenty-five years.[1]

Ironic, then, that thousands of years ago, the laid-back Romans and Greeks—who wrote on wax-coated tablets with a stylus made of metal, bone, or ivory—possessed an understanding of diabetes even though they had no blood tests for them. Though it may sound gross to modern sensibilities, the Romans and Greeks could detect diabetes by simply tasting a person's urine. *Yech!* Though I wonder who mastered this breakthrough (and especially how they did so), they discovered that some people's urine had a sweet taste, or *mellitus*—the Latin word for "sweet." In addition, the Greeks realized that when patients with sweet urine drank any fluids, they generally excreted these fluids in their urine almost as rapidly as they went in the mouth, similar to a siphon. In fact, the Greek word for "siphon" is *diabetes.* So now you know how we got the name *diabetes mellitus*: it all started by tasting the urine. I for one am glad that doctors abandoned this practice and that we can check a patient's blood sugar!

I have good news for you too: not only is this disease thousands of years old, but also so is God's power to heal. Just as God healed the sick thousands of years ago in the days of the Bible, He still heals today! He has also provided a wealth of proven biblical principles and invaluable medical knowledge about the human body. You can control the symptoms and potentially damaging effects of diabetes while you seek Him for total healing. You are destined to be more than a victim. You are destined to be a victor in this battle!

Your first order of battle in attacking the symptoms of diabetes, or prediabetes, is to know your enemy. After measuring its strengths, plan for ways you can defeat it. The enemy known as diabetes comes in many forms.

Different Types of Diabetes

Diabetes is actually a group of diseases including type 1 diabetes, type 2 diabetes, and gestational diabetes. Each type is characterized by high levels of blood sugar that is the result of either defective insulin production, defects in the action of insulin, or both.

A person does not just wake up one day with type 2 diabetes. Developing it is a slow, insidious process that usually takes years to a decade to develop. It always starts with prediabetes.

Prediabetes (formerly called *borderline* or *subclinical diabetes*) is a condition in which a person's blood glucose or hemoglobin A1c levels are higher than normal but not high enough to be diagnosed as diabetes. People with prediabetes have a greater risk of developing type 2 diabetes, heart disease, and stroke. From 2005 to 2008, based on fasting glucose or hemoglobin A1c levels, 35 percent of US adults had prediabetes. Applying this percentage to the entire US population in 2010 puts the estimate at 79 million adults with prediabetes.[2]

Diabetes is defined as a fasting blood sugar (FBS) level greater than or equal to 126 mg/dL or a casual blood sugar level (usually after eating) greater than or equal to 200 mg/dL. High blood sugar levels are usually accompanied by symptoms of diabetes, including frequent urination, excessive thirst, and changes in vision.[3]

In the past, type 1 diabetes was called insulin-dependent diabetes, juvenile-onset diabetes, or childhood-onset diabetes. Although it can strike at any age, this form usually occurs in children or young adults. In adults it is quite rare, with only approximately 5 percent of all cases of diabetes proving to be type 1 diabetes.[4]

While we do not have all the pieces of the puzzle for this type, risk factors may be genetic or environmental. Some researchers believe that the environmental trigger is probably a virus. Others believe the trigger may be ingesting protein from cow's milk, especially during infancy. In my book *Eat This and Live! for Kids*, Dr. Joseph Cannizzaro and I recommend increasing your child's intake of vitamin D, reducing intake of cow's milk, limiting or avoiding gluten, and avoiding all nitrates and nitrites to prevent type 1 diabetes.

What we *do* know about type 1 diabetes is that it is caused by the body's immune system attacking itself and eventually destroying the beta cells in the pancreas. The beta cells are the only cells in the body that make insulin, which is the hormone that regulates blood sugar. Patients with type 1 diabetes require insulin either by injection or by an insulin pump in order to survive.

Over the years, my patients with type 1 diabetes who have maintained the best blood sugar control have been those using an insulin pump. Newer insulin pumps have remote controls, making it much easier to control your blood sugar. In treating patients, I have discovered that dietary and lifestyle changes and nutritional supplements will usually lower insulin requirements in type 1 diabetics, but they will still require insulin. Once you begin such a program, it is necessary to monitor your blood sugar daily, adjust your insulin accordingly, and follow up with your physician on a regular basis.

The hemoglobin A1c test is the best way to monitor your blood sugar over the long run. Hemoglobin is a protein that carries oxygen in the blood. It is present inside the red blood cells that live only for about ninety 90 to 120 days. The hemoglobin A1c measures how much glucose has entered the red blood cells and become stuck to the hemoglobin, similar to a fly stuck to flypaper.[5]

If someone has a high blood sugar level throughout the day, more sugar will stick to the hemoglobin. If blood sugar is typically only slightly elevated during the day, less sugar will stick to the hemoglobin, and the hemoglobin A1c will be lower.

Most diabetes specialists recommend that diabetic patients strive to lower their hemoglobin A1c to 6.5 percent or less to prevent most of the complications of diabetes. They also recommend that patients check this blood test every three to four months. I personally try to get my diabetic patients hemoglobin A1c to around 6 percent or less because at this level, I find that they rarely ever develop severe complications.

Individuals battling with type 1 diabetes will greatly benefit from the nutritional information and biblical truths shared in this book. Continue to follow your doctor's advice, continue to take your insulin, and consult him or her before making any lifestyle or nutritional changes. In addition, determine to believe God—who created your pancreas—for a miraculous touch of healing power. The Word of God says, "For nothing is impossible with God" (Luke 1:37, NLT).

Remember that faith is not a feeling or an emotion, but a choice. Specifically ask the Lord to heal your pancreas and restore its ability to manufacture insulin. Jesus said in Mark 9:23, "All things are possible to him who believes," and in Mark 10:27, "For with God all things are possible."

Type 2 Diabetes

Type 2 diabetes was previously called non-insulin-dependent diabetes or adult-onset diabetes. That's because, historically, most people contracted the disease in their adult years. Sadly, our nation's taste for high-sugar, high-fat diets seems to have removed age barriers. In recent years the medical community has reported that this form of diabetes accounts for a growing number of juvenile cases. In adults, 90 to 95 percent of all diabetes cases are type 2 diabetes.[6] And, according to the National Institutes of Health, 1.9 million new cases of diabetes in people twenty and older were diagnosed in 2010.[7]

Type 2 diabetes is more of a genetic disease than type 1. However, as I mentioned in the previous chapter, although genetic makeup may have "loaded the gun," environmental factors like belly fat, poor diet, and lifestyle will "pull the trigger." Stop playing the blame game. Face your need to change. If you're in danger of developing diabetes or have crossed the line, recognize that losing belly fat, controlling your diet, and exercising regularly means you will probably never develop diabetes or can usually reverse it. Take heart from the major diabetes prevention study that revealed that lifestyle changes reduced developing diabetes by more than 70 percent of high-risk people who were over sixty years old.[8]

The majority of people who develop type 2 diabetes still produce insulin; however, the cells in their bodies do not use the insulin properly. This condition is known as insulin resistance. Over time, insulin resistance leads to prediabetes and type 2 diabetes.

For years I have explained to patients that insulin is like a key that unlocks the door to your cells. Type 2 diabetes is similar to having rusty locks on those cells. Every cell in your body needs sugar. The hormone insulin removes sugar from the bloodstream and binds to insulin receptors on the surface of the cells, similar to a key unlocking a lock and opening the door. The insulin opens the door to the cells (figuratively speaking) and allows sugar to enter.

However, in type 2 diabetics, the cells resist insulin's normal function. In other words, the key goes in to unlock the lock. But, just like a rusty lock, the insulin does not work as well. If you have ever tried to open an old, rust-encrusted lock, you will understand this analogy.

Insulin levels then begin to rise as your body needs more and more insulin to allow sugar to enter the cells. This is similar to jiggling a key over and over until it springs the rusty lock. That means an excessive amount of insulin is needed to keep blood sugar levels in the normal range. Eventually, as cells become more and more insulin resistant, higher insulin levels are unable to lower the blood sugar. The blood sugar rises higher and higher, meaning the individual develops prediabetes and eventually type 2 diabetes. What is scary is that patients with prediabetes usually don't exhibit any symptoms.

As this stage of insulin resistance worsens, a person will eventually develop prediabetes. People with prediabetes typically have impaired glucose tolerance (IGT), impaired fasting glucose (IFG), or both. Often they do not know they have prediabetes. And it typically takes years—sometimes even more than a decade—to progress from prediabetes into full-blown type 2 diabetes.

By the time people develop type 2 diabetes, they typically experience such bothersome symptoms as increased thirst, increased urination, frequent nighttime urination, blurred vision, or fatigue. Type 2 diabetes is typically associated with obesity (especially truncal, which refers to fat deposits in the torso and abdomen), increasing age, a family history of diabetes, physical inactivity, or a history of gestational diabetes. Race or ethnic heritage also plays a role in risk factors. American Indians, Hispanic Americans, African Americans, and some Asian Americans and Pacific Islanders have a higher chance of developing type 2 diabetes and its complications.

Insulin resistance is the main cause of type 2 diabetes. Though usually a manageable problem, it is complicated by the fact that truncal obesity is one of the most important factors leading to insulin resistance. Obese people with type 2 diabetes must decrease their belly fat by choosing low-glycemic foods. This means that type 2 diabetics require a diet that:

- Is low in refined processed starches, such as white rice, white bread, potatoes, and pasta
- Contains very little sugar

HIGH-FRUCTOSE CORN SYRUP: SUGAR IN DISGUISE

If you have diabetes, your doctor has undoubtedly told you how important it is to limit the amount of sugar in your diet. Although you know you need to choose your foods carefully, food manufacturers can be sneaky. One ingredient to be extremely wary of is the presence of one of sugar's many aliases: high-fructose corn syrup (HFCS).

HFCS is a blend of glucose and fructose. Glucose is the form of sugar in your blood that you monitor as a diabetic. Fructose is the primary carbohydrate in most fruits. Well, if it's from fruit, it's healthy, right? Not exactly. It is true that it's OK to consume small amounts of fructose because your body metabolizes it differently. As a result, it does not trigger your body's appetite control center. However, consuming large amounts sets you up for increasing belly fat and a fatty liver, insulin resistance, and eventually diabetes.

Since HFCS is common in thousands of commercial food and drink products, I highly recommend that you stick to the outer aisles at the grocery store, where you will find fresh produce, whole grains, and lean meats. Avoid the center aisles, where the highly processed foods, boxed convenience items, and sugar-laden treats live. Follow this commonsense approach, and you will be well on your way to avoiding the risk of consuming the "stealth" sugar that hides inside many packaged, processed products. Many researchers believe that America's excessive intake of HFCS is responsible for our diabetes epidemic.

How bad is it? HFCS represents 40 percent of calorie sweeteners added to foods and beverages and—until the advent in recent years of pure-sugar versions of various soft drinks—was the only sweetener of soft drinks in the United States. The average American consumes about 60 pounds a year of HFCS. "So what?" you shrug. You may take a more serious outlook when you realize that the liver metabolizes fructose into fat more readily than it does glucose. This means that consuming HFCS can lead to a non-alcoholic fatty liver, which usually precedes insulin resistance and type 2 diabetes.

Almost every product on the grocery shelves today contains both nutritional information and a list of ingredients. Too many people complain that they don't understand these labels or that it takes too much time to read them. If you are battling diabetes or prediabetes, it will be well worth your time to get educated. And when it comes to HFCS, here is a simple rule to follow: if HFCS is one of the first ingredients on the label, don't eat or drink it. Here is a sampling of foods high in HFCS:

- Soft drinks
- Popsicles
- Pancake syrup
- Frozen yogurt
- Breakfast cereals
- Canned fruits
- Fruit-flavored yogurt
- Ketchup and barbecue sauce
- Pasta sauces in jars and cans
- Fruit drinks that are not 100 percent fruit

Gestational Diabetes

Although acquired during pregnancy, gestational diabetes only occurs in about 2 percent of pregnancies. Gestational diabetes is due to the growing fetus and placenta secreting hormones that decrease the body's sensitivity to insulin, which can lead to diabetes.

If a woman develops gestational diabetes, it usually goes away after giving birth. Only 5 to 10 percent of women with gestational diabetes are found to have type 2 diabetes after giving birth. However, this form of diabetes increases a woman's risk of developing type 2 diabetes later in life. Studies show that 35 to 60 percent of women who developed gestational diabetes will develop type 2 diabetes within ten to twenty years after pregnancy.[9] Gestational diabetes occurs more frequently among African Americans, American Indians, and Hispanic Americans.

A caution: Don't take your presence in one of these groups as evidence that you bound for trouble. Still, it can be a signal that you need to pay closer attention to diet, exercise, and losing belly fat. Such advice can be repeated for everyone in our "couch potato" nation.

Chapter 3

SYMPTOMS AND LONG-TERM COMPLICATIONS OF DIABETES

L isten to your body" is an adage that many doctors pass along to their patients. Although this is not a foolproof method—especially considering my previous observation that someone with prediabetes won't necessarily notice any symptoms—you should pay attention to any warning signs that physical trouble is brewing. There are countless numbers of people lying in the cemetery who passed off chest pains or other obvious signs of heart trouble as indigestion. Or they didn't want to bother anyone or take the time to go to the doctor. Ignore your body, and you could soon be pushing up daisies.

As with most diseases, early detection of diabetes is crucial. Silent enemies sometimes inflict the most damage. Fortunately, for some people diabetes has telltale symptoms (note that these aren't restricted to age or gender).

Don't panic just because you have noticed one of these symptoms. Some may occur periodically simply because you drank too much liquid one night, ate some spicy food, or stayed up too late. However, if you experience one or more of these symptoms on a regular basis, make an appointment with your physician to get screened for

TYPE 1 DIABETES

- Frequent urination
- Unusual thirst
- Extreme hunger
- Unusual weight loss
- Extreme fatigue and irritability[1]

TYPE 2 DIABETES*

- Any of the type 1 symptoms
- Frequent infections
- Blurred vision
- Cuts/bruises that are slow to heal
- Tingling/numbness in the hands/feet
- Recurring skin, gum, or bladder infections[2]

---

* Sometimes people with type 2 diabetes have no symptoms.

diabetes and prediabetes. Then you can apply the truths in this book and in God's Word to the situation. Above all, don't give in to fear or apathy.

Treatable and Beatable

As with most diseases, serious health complications occur when someone with diabetes fails to do anything about this very treatable—and beatable—disease. The more serious complications of diabetes include diabetic retinopathy (the leading cause of blindness in the United States), diabetic neuropathy (a degeneration of peripheral nerves that leads to tingling, numbness, pain, and weakness usually in extremities such as the legs and feet), kidney disease, and atherosclerosis or arteriosclerosis. Arteriosclerosis is hardening of the arteries. Atherosclerosis is when arteriosclerosis occurs due to fatty deposits on the inner lining of the arterial walls. Approximately 44 percent of diabetics will develop atherosclerosis of the carotid arteries and in peripheral arteries. Diabetics are approximately two to five times at greater risk of a heart attack or coronary artery disease compared to nondiabetics. Also, approximately 20–25 percent will develop either impaired kidney function or kidney failure on average of eleven years after diagnosis.[3]

Proponents of eating meat often point to Genesis 9:3, where God gave mankind the freedom to consume meat. What these advocates fail to appreciate is that the average American's excessive consumption of meat, as well as carbohydrates, sugar, and fat, can cause numerous health problems. Diabetics—particularly those who fail to control their insulin and blood sugar levels through proper diet, exercise, and lifestyle choices—are much more prone to heart disease, heart attacks, kidney disease (a primary cause of death in diabetics), foot ulcers (usually due to poor blood supply), and peripheral nerve disease in the feet.

In what can only be called a burst of wishful thinking, most people with diabetes think that they will never develop long-term complications. They rationalize that they will surely have early signs and symptoms before they develop these terrible complications. Or they assume they will be able to take medications that will reverse the impact of the disease.

I tell my patients that diabetes is similar to a house infested with termites. When termites have been eating away at a home for long enough, one day when the homeowner tries to hang a picture on a wall, a gaping hole may suddenly appear. Or a door suddenly sticks, and when the homeowner pushes on the door, the frame caves in. Now, this does not happen immediately. Termite-inflicted damage takes months or even years to surface, but the impact is unmistakable.

Poorly controlled diabetes is a silent killer that works in a way similar to termites. After many years, sometimes decades, terrible health conditions suddenly begin to surface thanks to long-term diabetes. While medications can slow the process or control some of the symptoms, they usually do not get to the root of the problem. This makes Michael Pollan's observation in chapter 1 about America's "solution" of turning a disease into a lifestyle an apt commentary on the folly of our nation's approach to our health crisis.

Long-term elevation of blood sugar eventually damages and destroys the beta cells of the pancreas, which are the insulin-producing cells. Oxidative stress and chronic inflammation will also eventually damage and destroy the insulin-producing cells. The longer these processes go on (high blood sugar, chronic inflammation, and oxidative stress), the more beta cells will die so that eventually, when the number of beta cells is half of their original number, type 2 diabetes is then typically irreversible. That is why it is so important to identify prediabetes and type 2 diabetes and lower the blood sugar as well as the inflammation before permanent damage is done.

Diseases and Complications

According to the National Institutes of Health (NIH), diabetes contributes to the following diseases and health complications:

Vascular disease

Heart attacks

As plaque accumulates in the coronary arteries from diabetes, people are more prone to develop heart disease or suffer a heart attack. When many diabetics suffer a heart attack, because of damaged nerves, they may not experience the typical severe chest pain associated with heart attacks. Some actually experience silent heart attacks, feeling no pain at all.

Peripheral vascular disease

Individuals with poorly controlled long-term diabetes are also at a much greater risk of developing peripheral vascular disease (atherosclerosis of the peripheral blood vessels). Long-term elevated blood sugar eventually accelerates plaque formation in all arteries of the body. Peripheral vascular disease is plaque formation usually in the legs and feet. Many long-term diabetics can no longer feel their pulse in their feet, or they experience *claudication* (pain in the calves with walking that subsides with rest). Both of these are symptoms of peripheral vascular disease.

Long-term diabetics who smoke and have high cholesterol and high blood pressure are at a much greater risk of developing peripheral vascular disease. Fish oil, aspirin, and medications, along with aggressive risk factor modification, including blood sugar control, are usually needed to help people with peripheral vascular disease.[4]

Stroke

A stroke is sometimes termed a "heart attack of the brain." Since diabetics are prone to plaque buildup in the arteries that supply blood to the brain, this puts them at an increased risk of stroke. A diabetic may have a TIA (transient ischemic attack) in which he or she develops slurring of the speech, numbness, or weakness on one side of the body that usually goes away in less than five minutes. Having a TIA is an ominous sign of an impending stroke. If you experience this, go to the emergency room or see your physician immediately.[5]

Eye disease

Long-term diabetes also affects the eyes and may lead to a condition known as diabetic retinopathy. This is caused by damage to blood vessels in the retina, the tissue at the back of the inner eye, which converts light entering the eye into nerve signals sent to the brain. The long-term consequences: loss of vision and eventual blindness. Diabetic retinopathy is common among diabetics who have had the disease for more than ten years; between 40 and 45 percent of people with diabetes have some stage of diabetic retinopathy.[6] For the 2005–2008 time period, 4.2 million people with diabetes age forty or older had diabetic retinopathy. Of those, 655,000 had advanced retinopathy that could lead to severe vision loss.[7] Diabetic retinopathy is one of the leading causes of blindness.

Without good blood sugar control, numerous changes occur in the eyes that can be seen in the retina. Diabetes causes a weakening of the tiny blood vessels in the eyes, which may eventually rupture and form retinal hemorrhages. These hemorrhages can form clots that may eventually cause retinal detachment.

If you are diabetic, it is crucial that you get examined each year by an ophthalmologist. An ophthalmologist will examine your eyes and do a thorough screening for signs of retinopathy. He may decide to use laser surgery to save your vision. However, don't depend on this as a convenient way to correct vision problems. As a result of laser surgery, some people experience a minor loss of vision and a decrease in night vision. This is why it is critically important to maintain good blood sugar control to prevent diabetic retinopathy or to slow or stop its progression.

Kidney disease

In the United States, diabetes is the underlying cause of approximately half of the people who require long-term dialysis, as well as being the leading cause of kidney failure.[8] However, don't let these statistics scare you. The majority of people with diabetes *do not* develop kidney disease. Of those who do, most do not progress to kidney failure. This is good news. It means that even with diabetes, simply controlling your blood sugar will almost always prevent kidney disease.

Controlling your blood sugar and blood pressure, along with maintaining a healthy diet and losing weight, is critically important if you are facing the challenge of kidney disease. Your doctor may prescribe a medication such as an ACE inhibitor, and I recommend a form of vitamin B_6 (pyridoxal 5 phosphate), which also helps to protect the kidneys.

Early detection of kidney disease can help you avoid kidney failure. However, even regular urinalysis doesn't provide detection of the early stages of kidney disease. Therefore it is important to get a specific test for microalbumin, which can detect protein in the urine years before a regular urinalysis. Make sure your doctor checks the microalbumin level in your urine at least once a year.

Diabetic neuropathy

Long-term diabetes eventually affects the nervous system, which leads to a condition known as to diabetic neuropathy. Approximately 60 to 70 percent of diabetics have some form of peripheral nerve damage. This often affects the feet and hands, and the patient usually describes symptoms of numbness or decreased ability to feel light touch and pain.[9] They also usually develop burning and tingling sensations, or extreme sensitivity to touch. This is especially acute in the feet, and symptoms are usually worse at night.

Diabetic neuropathy may eventually lead to foot ulcers. Sometimes these ulcers become infected. If not treated promptly, they may lead to a severe infection and, eventually, amputation. Maintaining good foot care, wearing comfortable shoes and socks, careful daily inspections of your feet, and maintaining good blood sugar control are all important aspects of treating diabetic neuropathy.

I recommend to diabetic patients that they never go barefoot outdoors, and that those with diabetic neuropathy see a podiatrist or foot specialist regularly.

About 60 to 70 percent of people with diabetes have mild to severe forms of nervous system damage. This can cause impaired sensation or pain in the feet and hands, slowed digestion of food, carpal tunnel syndrome, or erectile dysfunction.[10] The majority of diabetic men over the age of fifty will experience the latter. However, if discovered early enough, this problem can be prevented or reversed through the loss of belly fat, controlling blood sugar with diet and exercise, stress reduction, and taking supplements and hormone replacement. Erectile dysfunction gets the attention of most men, and typically the greater the belly fat, the more severe the erectile dysfunction.

A condition called gastroparesis is when the muscles in the stomach do not function normally to move food through the digestive tract. This occurs when the vagus nerve is damaged. This usually causes slowed and impaired digestion, nausea, and vomiting. It also interferes with blood sugar levels and affects one's nutrition.

Amputations

In the United States more than 60 percent of non-traumatic, lower-limb amputations occur among people with diabetes. In 2006, about 65,700 lower-limb amputations were performed on people with diabetes.[11] The lower extremities are more susceptible to circulatory impairment caused by diabetes simply because they are farther from the heart. The nutrients and oxygen in the bloodstream must travel a greater distance through the blood vessels and capillaries to nourish cells in the feet and toes. You may think that is no big deal unless you consider that there are 25,000 miles of capillaries in the average adult's body.

Dental disease

Dental disease, particularly in the form of periodontal disease (a type of gum disease that can lead to tooth loss), occurs with greater frequency and severity among people with diabetes. Adults age forty-five or older with poorly controlled diabetes are nearly three times more likely to develop severe periodontitis than those without diabetes. The likelihood is even greater (4.6 times) among smokers with poorly controlled diabetes.[12]

Pregnancy complications

Poorly controlled diabetes prior to conception and during the first three months of pregnancy among women with type 1 diabetes can cause major birth defects in 5 to 10 percent of pregnancies and spontaneous abortion in 15 to 20 percent of pregnancies. During the second and third trimesters, if diabetes is not controlled, it can result in large babies, posing a risk to both mother and child.[13]

Other illnesses

In addition to the long list I just reviewed, diabetics are more susceptible to other illnesses. And they have a worse prognosis if they do come down with these illnesses. For instance, diabetics are more likely to die from flu and pneumonia than nondiabetics.[14]

Glycation

The main reason diabetics develop complications such as heart attacks, peripheral vascular disease, kidney disease, neuropathy, eye disease, and erectile dysfunction is because of the accumulation of AGEs (advanced glycation end-products). The higher the blood sugar and the longer the time the blood sugar is elevated, the more AGEs will accumulate. The sugar (glucose) molecule reacts with any free amino groups of proteins, lipids, and nucleic acids and forms AGEs. AGEs form cross links between proteins, which alter their structure and function.

AGEs are the root cause of almost all complications of diabetes, including retinopathy, neuropathy, nephropathy (kidney disease), and atherosclerosis. AGEs in tissues increase the rate of free radical production fifty times the rate of unglycated proteins. AGEs attach to LDL cholesterol, increasing oxidation of the cholesterol and leading to plaque in the arteries or atherosclerosis. They also accumulate in the kidneys, nerves, eyes (lens and blood vessels), brain (accelerating brain cell death), skin (forming wrinkles and sagging skin), blood vessels and nerves of the penis (accelerating erectile dysfunction), as well as in all muscles, organs, and tissues throughout the body.

AGEs are simply useless cellular trash or debris that eventually damages and destroys tissues and organs as they accumulate. They have no beneficial function at all and cannot be utilized for energy. Once they form, they are irreversible and cannot be repaired, detoxified, or removed from the body.

This is why long-term elevation of blood sugar is so dangerous. You are accelerating the aging process and accumulating cellular debris that will eventually impair and destroy many different tissues in the body as they accumulate. The higher the blood sugar, the more AGEs will accumulate, which literally invites a host of deadly diseases into your body and accelerates the aging process.

I wish people could comprehend that in a prediabetic or diabetic patient, that slice of cake, piece of pie, fudge, brownie, candy bar, or soda is raising the blood sugar and creating irreversible AGEs. The AGEs in turn are wrinkling your skin, causing erectile dysfunction in men, and setting you up for cardiovascular disease, kidney disease that eventually may require dialysis, and peripheral neuropathy, in which you may develop numbness and tingling or burning pains in your feet and extremities. Are you getting the picture?

Only you can start to make the correct choices. Marketers have glamorized sugary items, and oh, how attractive and enticing are the birthday cakes and pastries when you enter the bakery section of any grocery store as you inhale that wonderful aroma of freshly baked pastries. But then go to a dialysis unit where patients typically have to be dialyzed three times a week for three hours a treatment, and you will find the majority of those patients are diabetic.

There is a simple blood test to gauge your rate of AGE formation, and it's called the hemoglobin A1c test or HbA1c. I discussed briefly in chapter 2 about HbA1c. This is a very common test used to monitor a diabetic's blood sugar over a few months, but it can also monitor glycation in a prediabetic patient or even healthy patients without prediabetes or diabetes. I am amazed at how many of my (so-called) healthy weight patients have an elevated HbA1c and don't even realize it. They are eating desserts and drinking sodas, and because they are not overweight or obese, they think they are healthy. However, they are forming AGEs, which are accumulating and accelerating the aging process.

Hemoglobin is a protein inside the red blood cells (RBCs) that enables the RBCs to carry oxygen. However, the hemoglobin protein is also very prone to glycation. Glycation occurs easily to the hemoglobin when the blood sugar is elevated; the higher the blood sugar, the higher the percent of hemoglobin becomes glycated.

RBCs have a life span of approximately ninety days. I monitor my diabetics HbA1c every three to four months, and I typically see improvements in their HbA1c as they lose belly fat and as they exercise, follow a low-glycemic diet, and take a few supplements.

Most nondiabetic Americans have an HbA1c of 5.0 percent to 6.4 percent. If the HbA1c is greater than 6.5, the patient has diabetes. Approximately 70 percent of American adults have an HbA1c between 5.0 percent and 6.9 percent.[15]

What most people do not realize is that the HbA1c does not have to be 6.5 or higher to cause health problems. Every 1 percent increase in HbA1c, even when the HbA1c was in the normal range, was associated with an increased risk of heart attacks, cancer, and increased mortality.

I believe the optimum HbA1c is 5.0 percent or less since this is the normal rate of glycation. Quite a few diabetics have an HbA1c of 10, which is twice the normal rate of glycation. The higher the HbA1c, simply speaking, the faster you are aging.

After reading through these dismal complications, you may feel like young David when he stood before the 9-foot giant Goliath. *Caution: do not give in to fear!* These are the complications that most often affect diabetics whose blood sugar levels are not controlled through proper diet and exercise. But they do not mean you cannot find methods of coping with them and ultimately overcoming them.

In the face of these medical facts, your goal is to take advantage of the wealth of wisdom in God's Word and in the medical knowledge He has given us over the centuries. Wise choices can help you avoid these complications altogether. Most importantly, your primary goal is to take hold of the healing Jesus offers. Just as Jesus healed the woman with a seemingly incurable flow of blood (Matthew 9:19–22), He is able to heal today. Hebrews 13:8 says He is the same yesterday, today, and forever. Armed with this promise, you can move forward in the battle against diabetes, knowing that the Savior is bigger than any physical obstacle you are facing.

As you go, it will help to know some of the oft-hidden contributors to diabetes. The next four chapters will review these hidden factors.

Chapter 4

HIDDEN CONTRIBUTOR #1: CHRONIC STRESS AND ADRENAL FATIGUE

Forty-year-old Tammy followed a sensible diet, rarely eating sugar, high-glycemic carbs, or excessive fats; she also used proper portion sizes. She exercised five times a week for thirty minutes and even lifted weights twice a week. Despite this healthy life-style, she still tipped the scales at 50 pounds over her ideal weight. No matter what, she complained that she couldn't seem to shed the unnecessary pounds or get her blood sugar under control.

STRESS STATS

- Work-related stress may double your risk of dying from heart disease.

- Seventy-five to 90 percent of all doctor visits are prompted by stress-related ailments.

- Forty-three percent of adults deal with adverse health effects of stress.

- Stress is directly linked to the six leading causes of death (heart disease, cancer, lung ailments, accidents, cirrhosis of the liver, and suicide).

- Stress costs the American workforce more than $300 billion each year in lost work time, reduced productivity, and health-care compensation.[1]

After gently probing for details, it didn't take long to identify the source of her problem. It stemmed from all the "drama" in her life. A part-time secretary, Tammy cleaned houses on the side to earn extra spending money. Although her secretarial job only took part of her day, while at the office her boss ran her ragged. As a result, she suffered from tension headaches almost daily. Mix in her part-time job, and she rarely had time to her-self, since many after-work hours were consumed by carpooling three of her children to after-school activities such as dance lessons, ball practice, and piano lessons. This hectic pace also translated to habitual tardiness, which often left her upset and frustrated.

To add to the chaos, Tammy had an older son from a previous marriage who had hit a rebellious streak. Though only sixteen, he had already been arrested several times and made regular trips to the juvenile detention center. He frequently sneaked out of the house late at night to party with friends. In addition to getting drunk, he had been caught using drugs and regularly skipping school.

As you can imagine, Tammy's son's actions were also taking a toll. She had difficulty sleeping at night and worried throughout the day that police would call to inform her that her son was in jail again—or even dead. In addition, Tammy and her husband constantly argued over what to do with their rebellious son, which created more tension at home.

Despite a healthy diet and exercise, Tammy felt overwhelmed. She was literally in survival mode. Chronic stress had raised her cortisol levels so high it locked her into obesity. The same is true for millions of Americans living out-of-control, overloaded lifestyles. Any time you combine too many obligations, too much debt, and too many worries with an unhappy marriage, rebellious children, and sleep problems, you find disaster. Such loads are enough to keep people stressed out—and overweight—constantly!

Why? Excessive stress can increase glucose levels in the blood, promoting weight gain. For patients with diabetes, it's even worse, since this predisposes them to long-term complications—including kidney disease, eye disease, neuropathy, and vascular disease.

In one study, a group of diabetic patients participated in education sessions, both with and without stress management training. Such training included progressive muscle relaxation, breathing techniques, and mental imagery. All participants were at least thirty years of age and managing their diabetes with diet, exercise, and/or non-insulin medications.[2]

At the end of one year, 32 percent of the patients in the stress management group had hemoglobin A1c levels that were lowered by 1 percent or more. However, only 12 percent of the control subjects had hemoglobin A1c levels this much lower. As I stated in the previous chapter, hemoglobin A1c is a standard blood test used to determine average blood sugar levels over a period of a few months. Lowering hemoglobin A1c by 1 percent is considered highly significant; stress management did this in nearly one-third of the patients.[3]

Stress reduction is crucial in helping control diabetes since a high level of cortisol—the main stress hormone—is associated with increased belly fat, elevated blood sugar, and increased insulin levels. (I teach numerous stress-reduction techniques in my book *Stress Less*. I recommend that you consult this book for more information.)

The Stress Response

Our bodies trigger a stress response whenever we encounter a physical, mental, or emotional stressor, commonly known as "fight or flight." Walter

Cannon first described this response in 1915 after observing threatened animals whose sympathetic nervous systems experienced a discharge that prepared them to either stand and fight or flee.[4] Scientists soon realized this represented a common response among all vertebrates who face stress. More than one hundred years ago, most of our stressors were physical in nature—injury, danger, attacks, hard labor, and so on. However, today most stressors are emotional or psychological. They involve our perceptions and thoughts, showing how the definition for stress has changed.

When we encounter such stress, our heart rate increases, blood pressure rises, lungs breathe in more oxygen, pupils dilate, and the mind becomes extremely alert and focused. Blood is diverted away from the digestive tract and to our muscles so we can fight or flee. Our body dumps sugars and fats into the bloodstream to energize our body. While our immune function and digestion go on standby, all our other systems shift into high-alert mode. Adrenaline and cortisol, two powerful stress hormones, are then released into the body. Once the perceived stress or danger is over, both return to normal levels.

The problem is not when this occurs occasionally, but when unremitting stress causes frequent or prolonged activation of our stress response. Like a car's accelerator becoming stuck, our stress response gets stuck when it is repeatedly and routinely activated. It is not difficult to see why: with stress chemicals continually released into the bloodstream, the body stays in a perpetual state of high alert, continually spewing out stress hormones. This is comparable to your body burning ten dollars worth of energy for a two-cent problem. Over time, your body eventually is burned out similar to a car out of gas.

After a stressful event, our response is supposed to shut off, causing stress hormones to return to normal. This is called the recovery phase. Stress hormones are designed to save our lives in the short term. Yet when they are chronically released, they instead can threaten our lives. Many diseases are associated with problems adapting to stress. More commonly called "diseases of adaptation," these include heart disease and gastrointestinal disturbances such as acid reflux, ulcers, and irritable bowel syndrome. Elevated stress causes decreased immune function and frequent colds, flu, and sinus infections. It is also associated with high blood pressure, arrhythmias, tension headaches, allergies, and memory loss. Chronic stress may lead to anxiety and depression, which are commonly associated with weight gain and obesity. I am convinced that chronic stress is one of the main roots of our nation's obesity epidemic.

How Chronic Stress Makes You Fat

When your cortisol and adrenaline levels are chronically elevated, this causes stored sugar (known as glycogen) to be released from the muscles and liver into the bloodstream. This also causes the release of fat into the bloodstream to be used as energy. Fat and sugar are great when immediately burned for energy, but they cause weight gain when the body stores them. Unfortunately, the latter happens more frequently in society because of the shift in stressors from physical to psychological. The redefinition of stress has literally changed our country's shape. Since more individuals are emotionally and psychologically stressed, we naturally see more obese people.

Back in the "old days" of primarily physical stress responses, we would run or fight, burning off the sugars and fats released into our bloodstream. Now that most of our stress is psychological, we often stew in our stress juices. Instead of burning sugars and fats, we release more insulin, which causes more fat storage. It's a relatively simple equation: when cortisol levels rise, eventually insulin levels rise. Chronic stress raises cortisol, which eventually then raises insulin levels. The two work together as a "dynamic duo" of weight gain.

How ugly is this two-headed beast? Let me mention just a few of the ways one of these elements—cortisol—complicates the problem. Chronically elevated cortisol makes your body less sensitive to leptin, the hormone that tells your brain you are full. These high levels also stimulate the appetite, making you extremely hungry. At the same time, cortisol promotes the release of neuropeptide Y, a chemical in the brain that triggers a craving for carbohydrates. So far that's three negatives, each coming from a different angle. Not good.

> **EVERYDAY STRESS RELIEF**
>
> - De-clutter your house, office, car, etc.
> - Reevaluate and prioritize your deadlines.
> - Avoid unnecessary competition (i.e., finding the perfect parking spot, weaving through traffic).
> - Single-task more, multitask less.
> - Write (i.e., journaling can be a great way to release stress).

When you face a physical stressor, such as being attacked, your fight-or-flee response suppresses your appetite during the event. Following a trauma, increased cortisol levels will induce a bigger appetite. The same is true for psychological stress; after the trauma, your cortisol levels rise. Instead of helping you burn fat, however, high cortisol levels cause your metabolic rate to slow down. If you regularly get stressed out, your testosterone and DHEA levels also dwindle. Both of these valuable hormones not only assist in building muscle and burning fat, but they also help you cope with stress. To make matters worse, cortisol is the only hormone in the body that actually increases as you age.

Cortisol-Raising Foods

Although skipping meals is a prime offender for causing increased cortisol levels, several foods and beverages prompt the same response. Sugars, desserts, sodas, high-glycemic starches, and alcoholic beverages can raise both cortisol and insulin levels. Foods high in sugar spike the blood sugar, which usually causes the pancreas to secrete excessive insulin. This may also trigger hypoglycemia or low blood sugar. When this happens, the brain sends a signal to the adrenal glands to increase cortisol levels, which raises the blood sugar and raises insulin levels, setting the stage for prediabetes and eventually type 2 diabetes.

Caffeine will raise cortisol levels as well. Only 200 milligrams of caffeine, which is equivalent to one and a half to two cups of coffee, can raise cortisol by 30 percent within one hour. Now imagine what a grande Starbucks coffee with 550 milligrams of caffeine can do! And, when it comes to cortisol, sodas high in caffeine and sugar pose a double whammy. Foods that you are allergic to, or sensitive to, can also raise cortisol levels. So can herbal stimulants, such as guarana, bitter orange, and country mallow, and excessive intake of chocolate. Is your head swimming over all these "no-nos"? Live by a simple rule of moderate consumption of most food and avoiding sugars and high-glycemic foods, and you will be on your way to lowering cortisol and insulin levels and controlling your blood sugar.

Signs of Stress

Have you ever wondered why most people gain weight in the belly region? Draped over your stomach is the omentum, which is a sheet of visceral fat. It has receptors that bind to cortisol like magnets. When this union occurs, the omentum can store greater amounts of fat. Unfortunately, as this fat—the most toxic in the body—increases without being burned off, you become bubble wrapped with abdominal fat. With higher insulin and cortisol levels, you create a cycle that locks your body into becoming a fat production factory. The more belly fat, the more stress hormones are produced and released into the bloodstream, and the more fat is stored in the belly. To make matters worse, this not only promotes fat storage, but it also typically *prevents* the release of fat.

This frequently happens among people who are stressed out. Unfortunately, many stressed-out, overweight people add to their stress by worrying about gaining weight every time they eat. With this kind of outlook, meals are stressful experiences. (Remember, the majority of our stress is in perceptions.)

Another common condition of overstressed individuals is insulin resistance. Besides promoting fat storage in the abdomen, high cortisol levels cause the liver and muscles to release glycogen or stored sugar, which usually raises blood sugar and elevates insulin levels. Over time, cells may become insulin-resistant. When that happens, the body secretes more cortisol in an effort to balance the effects of excessive insulin. This produces more body and belly fat.

Adrenal Fatigue

Chronic stress, pain, illness, and injury, as well as anxiety and depression, can eventually take a toll on your adrenal glands. These two thumb-sized glands sit atop your kidneys, which manufacture stress hormones. When a stressor or stressors persist, these glands are unable to keep up with the production demands of the body, resulting in adrenal fatigue. After being stressed for years, the adrenal glands become weary and only produce a limited amount of stress hormones. This leaves a chronically stressed-out person with low levels of cortisol and DHEA, which also helps one to adapt to stress. Although high cortisol levels are associated with weight gain, so are low levels. The reason: individuals suffering from low levels are typically so "burned out" and fatigued they will not exercise. Their lack of activity further traps them into adrenal burnout or fatigue.

> **FUN ISN'T FRIVOLOUS**
>
> Modern life has more than its share of stress, whether that is too many deadlines, too much to do, a lack of free time…you can name the stresses that fill your life. That's why experts say that having fun isn't a dirty word. They recommend doing something you did as a child, such as playing with an electric train or playing at the park with your grandchildren.[5]

Adrenal fatigue is different from Addison's disease. The latter is adrenal failure, when the adrenal glands no longer function. In adrenal fatigue, the adrenal glands are able to make enough cortisol for life but not enough to enjoy good health. Unfortunately, many physicians fail to recognize or diagnose this disorder, even though it is becoming more prevalent.

There are actually three stages of adrenal fatigue, with stage 3 being the worst. (Refer to my book *Stress Less* for more information.[6]) The most common symptom of adrenal fatigue is low energy levels. People with adrenal fatigue will typically be extremely tired and sluggish. Cortisol levels typically peak between 6:00 and 8:00 a.m. and then gradually decline throughout the day until fading to their lowest levels at night.

Individuals suffering from severe adrenal fatigue start their days with their adrenal reserves drained and usually with low cortisol levels. They usually have problems sleeping and find it difficult to get out of bed in the morning. This means their energy dips severely in the early morning and usually again in the afternoon between 3:00 and 6:00 p.m. They usually feel good after about 6:00 p.m. and may get another boost in energy at 11:00 p.m. They work best late at night, and their best sleep is typically between 7:00 and 9:00 a.m. (and unless you're working an afternoon shift, you have to be at the office by then, or at least getting ready for work.)

Other symptoms of adrenal fatigue include weight gain, cravings for salt and salty foods, hypoglycemia (low blood sugar), and lack of stamina. Individuals with adrenal fatigue usually need to rest after emotional stress, often have a decreased sex drive, and suffer from environmental and food allergies, sensitivities, and lack of concentration. They may be nervous, irritable, or experience muscle weakness or frequent colds and infections (especially sinus infections). They tend to get light-headed when going from a lying to a standing position. Women suffering from this are prone to having PMS.

If you have many of these symptoms, you likely have adrenal fatigue and may need adrenal hormone testing. To find a physician who recognizes and treats adrenal fatigue, visit www.worldhealth.net.

How the Nervous System Responds to Stress

The autonomic nervous system, often referred to as the automatic nervous system, has two branches: the sympathetic and the parasympathetic. The sympathetic nervous system is responsible for the stress response, which can eventually lead to weight gain. The parasympathetic nervous system, on the other hand, is responsible for the relaxation response, which usually helps you to lose weight.

The key, then, is to learn how to turn off the chronic stress response, turn on the relaxation response, and eventually balance the stress response. Sound simple enough? I have written numerous books on this topic, including *Stress Less*, *Stress Management 101*, *Deadly Emotions*, and *The New Bible Cure for Stress*, all of which go into detail on coping with stress. Remember, most stress is based on our perceptions. If we learn to change our perceptions, we can usually flip the switch to the relaxation response.

One great way to change your perceptions is to take what I call the "six months to live" test. Imagine you only had six months to live. How would you live? What would you make a priority? What would you spend more time doing? Less time doing? I hope you would realize the need to slow down, decrease your stress, and learn to say no when people ask you to do something you do not want to do. Most people facing this daunting situation immediately decrease their obligations and spend more time with loved ones. If you knew you only had six months to live, you would likely do the same. You would probably forgive people—even the ones who hurt you—in order to find peace, love, joy, and happiness. You would overlook minor stressors and many major ones. With such a brief time to live, you would soon realize that most of your major stressors are actually minor.

You don't have to wait for a doctor to tell you that you have six months to live to initiate these changes. Almost all will result in an overall sense of peace and serenity, which brings rest to the body, soul, mind, and spirit. Since the mind holds our perceptions, can you see how changing perceptions is a key to transforming the other parts of your being? I believe following the Serenity Prayer is one of the best ways to begin to change perceptions: "God, grant me the serenity to accept the things I cannot change, courage to change the things I can, and wisdom to know the difference."

Tammy Deals With Stress

To draw some practical application, I will return to Tammy, the patient I told you about at the beginning of this chapter. After we identified the stressful elements in her life that were sabotaging weight loss and creating insulin resistance, we devised a plan for managing them. If you are in a similar situation, failing to cope with chronic stress means training your body for fat storage. Yet the good news is that stress can be managed. This is what most people (Tammy among them) do not realize.

Here are the steps I laid out for her. I hope that you can benefit from some by adapting and modifying them for your situation.

I had Tammy prioritize her activities, which made her realize that her children's well-being topped her list of desires. When she gave up her part-time housecleaning job, it freed up more time to spend with her children.

Tammy instituted margin into her life, which is breathing room. When she did so, she was no longer late to her children's activities. Ironically, her habitual tardiness had been sending the message to her children that they were unimportant. By allowing room for margin, she opened her eyes to their situations and feelings.

Tammy learned to say no. When she had been a "people pleaser," other coworkers pawned off their responsibilities onto Tammy. In effect, their stress became hers. I taught her to be assertive and say, "No, unfortunately I cannot fit that into my schedule." This made a world of difference in her energy levels, attitudes, and relationships.

Tammy added a twice-weekly yoga class to her exercise schedule. I also made sure that her aerobic workouts were in her fat-burning heart-rate range, which helped her to burn off excessive stress chemicals, sugars, and fats.

To deal with tension headaches, I taught Tammy breathing exercises and progressive muscle relaxation techniques. She soon discovered that they could help relieve headaches.

Tammy's greatest stress was her rebellious son. Because this was somewhat out of her control, I placed Tammy on an herbal adaptogen combination to help her cope and the amino acid L-tryptophan to help her sleep.

Eventually Tammy and her husband agreed to send her son to a military-type boarding school that separated him from negative peers and taught him discipline. With her marriage restored, Tammy could relax.

When Tammy's stress responses relaxed, the weight literally melted away. That almost sounds too simple, but it's true. She lost 50 pounds in less than eight months with no extraordinary effort. She did not change her diet or exercises, other than adding yoga and working out in her fat-burning heart-rate range. To add to the happy ending, when her son visits at holidays, he is respectful, loving, and appreciative. Peace finally reigns in Tammy's home.

If you are stuck in obesity and deal with chronic stress or adrenal fatigue, you can break free and live a healthier life too. It may be as simple as incorporating a few everyday practical tips to reduce stress, or it may require several stress-reduction techniques along with adaptogenic herbs. However, recognize that you do not have to follow the crowd drifting into obesity, prediabetes, and diabetes. You can turn off a stressful, overweight lifestyle and turn on a healthy, energetic, trimmed-down you.

Chapter 5

HIDDEN CONTRIBUTOR #2: COMPROMISED METABOLISM AND INSULIN RESISTANCE

I t's test time."

When the teacher or professor announced that, did you break out into a cold sweat? Feel butterflies dancing around your stomach? Regret that you rarely opened the textbook during the semester? Or have you banished all memories of test-taking to the hidden recesses of your mind? Do you hire an accountant to complete your income tax return—just so you won't have to fill out forms that remind you of the Florida Comprehensive Assessment Test (FCAT)?

While you may still get the chills over the idea of tests, in the fight to reverse diabetes it helps to memorize some basic information. Don't think of it as cramming for an exam that you can forget about next week; think of it as crucial data that will help you survive this dreaded disease. Understanding and retaining information about foods with low and high glycemic index values will help guide your day-to-day dietary choices and guide you in the direction of better health.

Let's start with a look at some of the commonly eaten foods—even so-called healthy ones—that contain extremely high glycemic index values. A high value is seventy or greater. Pure glucose or sugar dissolved in water (which is obviously not too healthy) has a glycemic index value of 100, which you might expect. But did you know buckwheat pancakes check in at an even higher rating of 102? Or that jasmine white rice is a hefty 109? That means these foods will raise your blood sugar faster than drinking pure sugar water! In addition, Fruit Roll-Ups has a glycemic index value of 99, just a smidgen below sugar water. Instant potatoes score a not-too-healthy 88. A single slice of Wonder bread registers at 73, meaning that white-bread sandwich you gulp down for lunch is high glycemic.

Eating these foods is similar to drinking sugar water since they all spike the blood sugar. Over time this can lead to truncal obesity, followed by insulin resistance or prediabetes. This may lead to metabolic syndrome and eventually type 2 diabetes. To decrease the chances of this happening, avoid sodas, alcohol, sugar-laden coffees, and even fruit juices. It is also important to avoid trans fats and decrease your consumption of foods rich in omega-6 oils, such as salad dressings, sauces, doughnuts, pastries, cake icing, and most fried foods, cooking oils, and crackers.

According to the University of Maryland Medical Center, the typical American diet tends to contain fourteen to twenty-five times as much omega-6 fatty acids as omega-3. While omega-6 acids are necessary for good health, a better balance is desirable. This is why the university gives a thumbs up to the Mediterranean diet with less meat (which is typically high in omega-6 fats and saturated fats) and emphasizes foods rich in omega-3s, such as whole grains, fresh fruits and vegetables, fish, olive oil, and garlic.[1] In addition, realize that trans fats and excessive intake of omega-6 oils also *cause* insulin resistance. On the other hand, omega-3 fats such as salmon and other fatty fish, as well as fish oil supplements, *decrease* insulin resistance.

If you have three or more of the five criteria mentioned in the sidebar Defining Metabolic Syndrome, then you have metabolic syndrome and are at a high risk of developing type 2 diabetes, heart disease, and truncal obesity. And those with truncal obesity are at a greater risk of developing insulin resistance or prediabetes, metabolic syndrome, and eventually type 2 diabetes. The National Heart, Lung, and Blood Institute says about 25 percent of American adults have metabolic syndrome.[3] Not only is this trend increasing at an alarming rate, but it is also expected to continue as the US population ages and becomes more obese.

Excessive consumption of saturated fats can also lead to insulin resistance.

DEFINING METABOLIC SYNDROME

Metabolic syndrome is closely associated with insulin resistance and truncal obesity and is simply a cluster of medical conditions that occur together. A commonly used definition of metabolic syndrome includes the following prerequisites:

- Abdominal obesity, defined as a waist circumference greater than 40 inches for a man and 35 inches for a woman.
- Elevated fasting serum triglycerides levels of 150 mg/dL or greater or drug treatment for elevated triglycerides.
- Low serum HDL (less than 40 mg/dL in males and less than 50 mg/dL in females) or drug treatment for low HDL.
- Hypertension, or a blood pressure greater than 130/85 mmHg, or drug treatment for hypertension.
- Fasting blood sugar greater than 100 mg/dL or drug treatment for elevated blood sugar.[2]

This includes such fatty meats as sausage, bacon, hamburger, pepperoni, and hot dogs, as well as dairy foods such as cheese, butter, and whole milk. In addition, large portion sizes can cause insulin resistance. It's important to observe proper portion sizes—with the correct fuel mixture of proteins, good fats, and low-glycemic carbohydrates—at each meal and with snacks to correct insulin resistance.

If you already know you have type 2 diabetes, metabolic syndrome, prediabetes, or truncal obesity, you will usually need to restrict starches even more. You will want to choose low-glycemic carbohydrates in place of refined starches and even limit your consumption of whole-grain, high-fiber starches. I counsel patients dealing with belly fat and insulin resistance to avoid most starches after 3:00 p.m., except for beans, peas, lentils, or legumes. These starches are high in soluble fiber, which helps to reverse insulin resistance. However, I advise limiting these late-day exceptions to one serving, which is only a half-cup—about the size of a tennis ball.

Insulin Resistance

Eating the right foods and limiting your intake is only part of the battle. As I mentioned previously, chronic stress creates an ongoing elevation in cortisol levels, which causes the body to continue releasing sugar into the bloodstream. As this occurs, insulin levels rise, blood sugar lowers, and the insulin simultaneously causes the body to store more fat. Not only does chronic stress start this "sugar cycle," but it also affects our food choices. Once caught in it, you are more likely to crave high-sugar beverages and high-glycemic foods. Skipping meals can also trigger this cycle, which creates a perfect setup for gaining more weight. Eventually this programs the body to resist insulin.

Insulin resistance occurs when the body's cells and tissues no longer respond normally to insulin. Insulin is an anabolic (or tissue-building) hormone that helps to build muscle tissue, but it also promotes the formation and storage of more fat. Essentially, the more insulin you secrete, the more weight—particularly belly fat—you will usually gain. To quickly review a section of chapter 2, insulin is like a key that opens the door to each cell so that

FROM DRINKS TO DIABETES

Researchers have discovered that people who consume one or more soft drinks a day are 48 percent more likely to develop metabolic syndrome than those who average less than one drink a day.[4]

sugar can enter into that cell. Much of the food that you eat is first converted to sugar and then arrives at the door of a cell in the form of blood sugar.

When your insulin is functioning effectively, it figuratively unlocks the door by binding to the insulin receptors on the surface of the cell. These receptors let the sugar in, which is then used to produce energy or build tissue.

Normally, sugars and highly refined, quickly digested carbohydrates convert to glucose and rapidly raise the blood sugar. The pancreas responds just as quickly by releasing large amounts of insulin to lower the blood sugar. This can go on for years without a person developing obesity, heart disease, prediabetes, or type 2 diabetes. However, after continuous consumption of these kinds of foods over many years, one's cells can become more resistant to insulin. As blood sugar continues to rise, the pancreas keeps churning out more insulin to lower the blood sugar and drive the sugar inside the cells. These elevated insulin levels then program the body for more fat storage, especially in the abdominal area. The higher the insulin levels in the blood, the greater the chance of storing belly fat—which, unfortunately, is the hardest fat to lose.

A Gradually Growing Disease

While type 2 diabetes is a hot topic and frequently mentioned in health news, it is important to realize you don't just wake up one morning with this condition. Type 2 diabetes develops over an extended period of time before doctors discover it. It begins with a diet high in sugars and highly refined carbohydrates. This eventually leads to weight gain and then insulin resistance or prediabetes, which can ultimately lead to metabolic syndrome and possibly type 2 diabetes. What these three conditions—prediabetes, metabolic syndrome, and type 2 diabetes—have in common is insulin resistance.

There are varying degrees of insulin resistance. To discover the extent of insulin resistance, have your physician perform a fasting blood sugar test. This test, which measures your blood glucose level, is usually done in the

CAUSE AND EFFECT

According to the American Diabetes Association, diabetes is now:

- The leading cause of kidney failure, accounting for 44 percent of cases in 2008

- Responsible for a heart disease death rate two to four times higher among diabetics than adults without diabetes

- The leading cause of new blindness cases among people ages twenty to seventy-four

- Responsible for more than 60 percent of non-traumatic, lower-limb amputations

- Responsible for mild to severe forms of nervous system damage in 60–70 percent of all diabetics[5]

morning after fasting all night, but it can be administered anytime after not eating anything for at least eight hours. If your FBS is greater than or equal to 100 mg/dL, you have insulin resistance and prediabetes.

In general, the higher your fasting blood sugar, the greater your insulin resistance. On the lower end of the scale is prediabetes, which is when your fasting blood sugar is between 100 and 125 mg/dL. Anything beyond this (126 mg/dL or greater) is considered type 2 diabetes.

Type 2 diabetes is the worst type of insulin resistance. Insulin resistance does not always lead to type 2 diabetes, but every type 2 diabetic is insulin resistant. The most common form, type 2 diabetes is also increasing to epidemic proportions. A study by the Centers for Disease Control and Prevention found a 49 percent increase in diagnosed diabetes in Americans from 1991 to 2001, which parallels a 61 percent increase in obesity during the same time period.[6] Studies project that the number of diagnosed diabetics in the United States will increase by 165 percent and reach an astronomical twenty-nine million people by the year 2050.[7]

Though some people with type 2 diabetes do not experience any prior symptoms, typical early signs include excessive thirst, frequent urination, excessive hunger, unexplained weight gain, and fatigue, especially after lunch or dinner. Fortunately, these individuals who experience such signals can usually lose weight fairly easily through a regimen of low-glycemic foods, moderate portion sizes, and regular exercise.

Reversing Insulin Resistance

To return to my opening reference to test-taking, the most important way to reverse insulin resistance is by choosing low-glycemic foods instead of moderate- or high-glycemic foods. Avoid sugars, sugary foods, and refined carbohydrates such as white bread, white rice, instant and regular potatoes, chips, crackers, and the like. It is also crucial that you eat more vegetables (especially those high in soluble fiber) and natural foods.

Type 2 diabetics and people with significant belly fat may require more extreme measures. Why? They are often severely metabolically compromised *and* severely insulin resistant. If you fall into either of these categories, you may need to decrease your starch intake even more—possibly cutting out starches and fruits altogether for a while in order to resensitize your insulin receptors. Avoid corn, rice, wheat, and other grains as well as potatoes, yams, pasta, bread, crackers, bagels, and pretzels until your body corrects its insulin resistance. While doing this, however, remember to consume adequate non-starchy vegetables, such as broccoli, green beans, salads, asparagus, and spinach. In addition, you may need to be monitored regularly by a diet counselor, nutritionist, or registered dietitian who can monitor your food journal and assist with meal planning.

Burn Off That Belly Fat!

Another crucial part of reversing insulin resistance is physical activity, which includes aerobic and strengthening exercises. While your eating program will concentrate on making sure you consume the right types of food, activity focuses on burning off fat (which in the case of insulin-resistant individuals is usually belly fat) and building muscle. We burn much of our glucose for energy in our muscle cells, especially in the arms and legs. However, as the number and size of fat cells increase, muscle cell volume typically decreases. This in turn decreases the number of insulin-binding sites, which programs the body for insulin resistance.

I typically have patients with insulin resistance exercise five or six days a week for at least thirty minutes a day. If a person has metabolic syndrome or type 2 diabetes, I may increase the length of their daily aerobic exercise to forty-five to sixty minutes, again for five or six days a week. I also place all patients with metabolic syndrome and type 2 diabetes on a strengthening program so they can build more muscle tissue to increase their number of insulin-binding sites. Often these patients are better off

THE NOT-SO-GOOD OL' AMERICAN DIET

A person who eats the typical Western diet of red meat, fried foods, and refined grains each day has an 18 percent greater chance of developing metabolic syndrome than someone else whose diet is dominated by fruits, vegetables, fish, and poultry.[8]

getting a personal trainer, both for the sake of accountability and to design an exercise program specific to their unique needs.

One of the main goals in reversing insulin resistance is to reduce your waist measurement. On the list of priorities for reversing diabetes, lowering waist size ranks higher than weight loss. As I've already explained, the abdominal region becomes a storehouse for toxic fat. This is especially true for type 2 diabetics, who need to make shedding belly fat a priority. For optimal health, a man should strive to get his waist measurement to less than forty inches, while a woman should aim for an initial goal of less than thirty-five inches.

Along with specific diet and exercise programs, it is critically important for insulin-resistant individuals to take certain nutritional supplements in order to resensitize the cells' insulin receptors. Supplements can often pinpoint areas that regular eating or exercising cannot. Important supplements for carbohydrate metabolism include cinnamon, chromium, lipoic acid, B vitamins, and omega-3 fats. Since the refining process for most white breads, white rice, and other refined foods means they have lost most of their fiber and nutrient content, these foods usually lack the valuable nutrients for optimal carbohydrate metabolism. Eating these nutrient-poor foods over the long term may eventually lead to nutrient deficiencies, which can contribute to greater insulin resistance. That is why the supplements listed above, plus a good multivitamin, are all important in rejuvenating and resensitizing the insulin receptors to help reverse insulin resistance.

Overcoming the Epidemic

Processed foods are taking a toll on the United States, whose residents have become addicted to sugars and highly refined carbohydrates. Any health practitioner, nutritionist, or dietician can draw a straight line between these habits and the obesity epidemic. Despite high levels of education and ever-increasing access to information via smartphones, the Internet, and other electronic tools, the average person is lost in the maze of information. Plodding along, stuck in lifelong familial and cultural habits, men and women alike can get easily locked into a lifestyle of eating zero-nutrition foods. After reading this, I hope you can see the connection between all these elements and the rise of insulin resistance, which has reached epidemic levels.

Correcting the problem starts with your diet. Such everyday foods as white breads, crackers, bagels, pretzels, chips, white rice, potatoes, instant oatmeal, most cereals, and sodas are not only part of the average American's diet, but they are also some of the main culprits behind developing insulin resistance. Trans fats, excessive saturated fats, and excessive omega-6 fats also contribute to insulin resistance and are equally common in salad dressings, fried foods, most dairy, processed meats and fatty cuts of meats, and sauces. Everywhere you look in America, there are large portion sizes. All of these have contributed significantly to the national surge of insulin resistance. You deserve a break today from this unhealthy glut of harmful substances. Pass the good health test by paying more attention to the fat, sugar, and sodium content of your diet. It will make a difference: just as the consequences of diabetes build over time, wise eating will bring long-term benefits. Just be patient!

The second main reason for our nation's epidemic of insulin resistance is our lack of physical activity. We have become a society of couch potatoes. With age and inactivity, we are losing valuable muscle mass, which is programming us for insulin resistance. And because of our inactivity, we are developing toxic belly fat. This not only worsens insulin resistance, but it also programs us for more belly fat.

These three elements—poor diet, lack of exercise, and increasing belly fat—make up the vicious cycle that has locked millions of Americans into insulin resistance, weight gain, and eventually prediabetes, metabolic syndrome, or type 2 diabetes. Many people have given up and are turning to fad diets, medications, and even lap-band surgery and other methods to help them lose weight. You don't have to do this! Not only are these alternatives (particularly surgery) expensive, but they can also pose health risks. By simply making a few changes in your lifestyle, over time you can resensitize your insulin receptors, open the door to weight loss, and lower your blood sugar.

Chapter 6

HIDDEN CONTRIBUTOR #3: INFLAMMATION, FOOD ALLERGIES, AND FOOD SENSITIVITIES

After the past decade, the American Southwest could be renamed the Burning Region. Of more than two dozen major wildfires in North America since 2002, nearly 60 percent have occurred in such states as California, Nevada, New Mexico, and Arizona.

It started with the largest fire in Sequoia National Forest history in California 2002. Other blazes in the Southwest followed that killed people, burned millions of acres, destroyed thousands of homes, and caused billions of dollars worth of damage. When the largest fire in Arizona's history struck in the summer of 2011, it destroyed more than 700 square miles of land and spread into New Mexico.[1]

Every fall it seems some state in this region is bracing for another string of wildfires, hoping the winds won't blow too hard and cause the fires to spread. I remember flying over California in the autumn of 2007. I looked out my window and saw separate fires smoldering almost everywhere. It is a moment I would describe as a Salvador Dali painting come to life.

This same surreal picture describes the blazes that are rampantly burning inside many Americans. However, unlike the Southwestern fires that hold the nation's attention for weeks on end, most of us are completely unaware of what is aflame. Sadly, this fire—systemic inflammation—continues to wreak havoc on millions of people, leading many toward further obesity.

What does inflammation have to do with weight gain and diabetes? I want to explain their close association and examine various dietary ways that can help you curtail this inflammation.

Chronic Inflammation and Disease

Inflammation is an important component of the immune system. It is essential for the healing process, since it is a programmed response, necessary for fighting infections and repairing damaged tissues. For example, when you sprain your ankle or develop tonsillitis, your white blood cells release chemicals into affected tissues. That prompts an increase in blood flow to the area, which causes redness, warmth, and pain. That is the reason your ankle or tonsils swell, become sore, and turn red. It's also why those areas heal faster. Without this response, wounds and infections may never heal. Eventually, that would put your entire body at risk.

However, problems arise when this inflammatory reaction becomes systemic and goes unchecked for months or years. When this happens, the same chemicals used for healing can cause weight gain and eventually trigger a host of deadly diseases.

Localized inflammation is easy to spot and feel. Its signs include swelling, redness, warmth, and pain. When the body triggers this healing response, you feel the pain of a strained muscle, a sprain, tendinitis, or bursitis. However, since systemic inflammation does not normally provide these symptoms, it goes unrecognized. Worse, when it is finally diagnosed, doctors and patients often dismiss it as a mere sign of aging or obesity. Unfortunately, this oversight often leads to further weight gain and disease.

While chronic inflammation is a symptom of virtually every disease, it also aggravates the disease. Unremitting inflammation brings exposure to inflammatory cytokines, which are destructive, cell-signaling chemicals that contribute to most degenerative diseases. Among them are atherosclerosis, heart disease, cancer, arthritis, metabolic syndrome, Alzheimer's disease, allergies, asthma, ulcerative colitis, Crohn's disease, hepatitis, celiac disease, and of course, diabetes.

You'll notice that almost all of these diseases are linked to obesity. Essentially, as Americans get fatter, chronic systemic inflammation increases and leads to many of these diseases. It also causes our bodies to age rapidly, including developing wrinkles.

Fat Feeds Inflammation

The obesity and inflammation connection is cyclical in nature: obesity causes increased inflammation, and increased inflammation causes more weight gain. This is partially due to fat cells manufacturing various types of inflammatory mediators, including interleukin-6, tumor necrosis factor-alpha, and plasminogen activator inhibitor-1. These all increase inflammation and are associated with atherosclerosis, or hardening of the arteries. Fat cells also produce the aforementioned cytokines. These are proteins that trigger the production of more inflammatory mediators, such as C-reactive protein (CRP). CRP is just one inflammatory marker that doctors use to measure the body's inflammatory state. If there is inflammation anywhere in the body, CRP typically increases. The CRP level rises in cases of chronic infection, elevated blood sugar (insulin resistance), and in overweight and obese people, especially among those with increased belly fat. Elevated CRP is also associated with an increased risk of both heart attack and stroke.

When the body produces more inflammatory mediators, such as CRP, this in turn sparks chronic systemic inflammation. Essentially, the more fat you have (particularly belly fat), the more inflammation you suffer.

Most people think of fat tissue as inactive, but that is far from the truth. Fatty tissue or fat storage areas, such as belly fat, are active endocrine organs that produce numerous types of hormones, such as resistin (which increases insulin resistance), leptin (which decreases appetite), and adiponectin (which improves insulin sensitivity and helps to lower blood sugar). The more fat cells, the more estrogen, cortisol, and testosterone your body produces. This is one of the reasons obese men typically develop breasts and obese women often grow hair on their face. Their fat cells are manufacturing more estrogen and testosterone, respectively.

When your fatty tissues spew out all these hormones—most likely raising your estrogen, testosterone, and cortisol levels—and produce tremendous inflammation in your body, the result is weight gain. Your extra toxic belly fat then sets the stage for type 2 diabetes, heart disease, stroke, cancer, and a host of other diseases. That's because belly fat is like those Southwestern wildfires I mentioned earlier. It spreads throughout your body and inflames your cardiovascular system, which causes the production of plaque in your arteries and inflammation in the brain. This can even potentially lead to Alzheimer's disease.

> **GOING LOW GLYCEMIC**
>
> A recent study of the Dutch population found that by lowering the glycemic index value of overall food intake by an average of ten points, participants decreased their CRP levels by 29 percent. Participants who continued on a low-glycemic diet also had higher levels of good cholesterol, improved insulin sensitivity, and reduced chronic inflammation—all of which indicated a decrease in risk of metabolic syndrome and cardiovascular disease.[2]

The Proof Is in the Fat

Several studies show the parallels between inflammation and fat. One study found that inflammation increased more than 50 percent in obese women whose fat was primarily in their hips and thighs. Among women with abdominal obesity, that number rose to a staggering 400 percent.[3]

A quick review may help you better understand the fat-inflammation connection. Every pound of stored fat requires about a mile's worth of blood vessels to sustain itself. In order to exist, fat cells secrete hormone-like substances to increase blood vessel growth. These blood vessels are supposed to nourish and feed accumulated fat. However, when the blood vessel growth cannot keep up with expanding fat, the fat cells become deprived of oxygen. These oxygen-deprived cells then release more inflammatory mediators to trigger more blood vessel growth...and on it goes. The wildfire spreads, made worse when the spark comes from belly fat, the most flammable source.

Other studies underscore the fact that inflammation not only *prepares* the body for adding additional fat but also even *precedes* this process. Two studies, the Atherosclerosis Risk in Communities Study and the Healthy Women Study, found higher concentrations of CRP and fibrinogen before weight gain occurred.[4] (Fibrinogen is a protein in the blood that, when elevated, can lead to blood clots or an increased risk of heart attacks and strokes.) Further research from Sweden showed that the higher the number of elevated inflammatory proteins, the greater the chances of weight gain.[5] Prior to these reports, experts assumed that obese people had higher levels of inflammatory proteins because of the cytokines their fatty tissues secreted. In other words, doctors thought that obese individuals continued to deal with greater inflammation because they were obese. Instead, these studies proved the other way was equally true: the higher the inflammatory proteins, the greater the odds of weight gain.

Without a doubt, fat deposited in the abdominal area leads to the greatest amount of inflammation. Conversely, when you decrease your body's inflammatory response, you will also lower your weight and your waist size. Given this situation, it is helpful to know which foods can trigger inflammation and which ones help control it.

A Deadly By-Product of the Western Diet: Inflammation

One of the biggest problems with our modern, high-fat, highly processed, high-sugar, high-sodium diets is that it has thrown off the balance in our bodies between inflammatory and anti-inflammatory chemicals called *prostaglandins*. Normally inflammation is a good thing that works to repair an injury or fight off infection in the body. It puts the immune system on high alert to attack invading bacteria or viruses to rid our body of these intruders, or in the case of an injury, it rushes white blood cells to the cut, scrape, sprain, or broken bone to promote healing and remove cellular debris or attack infections to facilitate healing. This is the good side of inflammation and an extremely important function of the immune system's small agents. When our bodies are in such an emergency, there is a complicated process through which more pro-inflammatory prostaglandins are created than anti-inflammatory ones, and the immune system responds to the sounding of this alarm. When the crisis is over, the balance swings in the anti-inflammatory direction and eventually balances out again.

If you look at this process in a grossly simplified sense, you will see that prostaglandins are produced from the foods we eat in an ongoing cycle, and each of the foods we eat has either a pro-inflammatory tendency or an anti-inflammatory one. Fatty acids are at the center of this. Omega-6 fatty acids are "friendly" to the creation of pro-inflammatory prostaglandins, and omega-3 fatty acids are "friendly" to the creation of anti-inflammatory prostaglandins. A more natural, Mediterranean-type diet will have a balance of pro- and anti-inflammatory-friendly foods; however, our modern high-fat, high-sodium, high-sugar, highly processed Western diet throws that balance off in favor of the production of pro-inflammatory prostaglandins.

Experts tell us that our typical US diet has doubled the amount of omega-6 fatty acids we consume since 1940 as we have shifted more and more away from fruits and vegetables to grain-based foods and the oils produced from them. In fact, we eat about twenty times more omega-6s than we do the anti-inflammatory omega-3s. Most of the animals we obtain food from today are also grain fed, so most of our meats, eggs, and dairy products are higher in omega-6s than they were a century ago. Also, as most of the fish in our stores are now farm raised, they are growing up on cereal grains instead of the algae and smaller fish they would live on in the wild, so even our fish are more sources of omega-6s than they used to be. Noting all of this, it is not hard to see why diseases caused by chronic systematic inflammation have grown to be such a problem in the Western world today.

Furthermore, essential fatty acids (EFAs) like omega-3 and omega-6 cannot be manufactured in the body and must be consumed either through diet or supplements. EFAs help the body repair and create new cells. In addition to reducing inflammation, omega-3 fatty acids can actually create special roadblocks in the body, making it harder for cancer cells to migrate from a primary tumor to start new colonies. Cancers that remain localized in one place are much easier to treat than those that metastasize (spread throughout the body).[6]

Because of the high omega-6 content of our diets, our bodies find more material for pro- than anti-inflammatory prostaglandins. Over time the natural, ongoing creation of prostaglandins will tip the balance toward systematic inflammation as more pro-inflammatory prostaglandins are produced than anti-inflammatory ones. Despite the absence of an actual emergency, this imbalance still sets off alarms calling for inflammation, and the immune system will respond accordingly. However, with no actual threat present, the immune system will start attacking things it normally wouldn't. This immune hypersensitivity can lead to a glut of problems ranging from simple allergies and weight gain to cancer, Alzheimer's disease, cardiovascular disease, diabetes, arthritis, asthma, prostate problems, and autoimmune diseases.

Many of these happen because as the immune system stays on high alert longer than it should, its agents begin to fatigue and make bad decisions, possibly leading to autoimmune disease or not destroying mutated cells, leading to cancer formation with more frequency. This can easily give way to cancer getting a foothold it won't easily relinquish.

Omega-3 fatty acids are clearly incredibly beneficial. Here are some omega-3 foods to include in your diet: raw nuts (almonds, walnuts), flaxseeds and flaxseed oil, fish (salmon, sardines, halibut, tongol tuna, herring, and cod), and fish oil. Obviously, it's important to know which fats to eat and which ones to avoid when it comes to preventing those harmful prostaglandins I mentioned above.

So, while using an understanding of the Mediterranean diet as a foundation, within that framework you should also look how pro-inflammatory or anti-inflammatory the foods you eat are as well. If you are having problems with allergies or the like, by eating more anti-inflammatory foods than pro-inflammatory ones, you can tip your balance back in the right direction.

One way to check your degree of inflammation is to have a C-reactive protein blood test. C-reactive protein is a promoter of inflammation and also a blood marker of systemic inflammation. Once you reach forty years of age, annual CRP testing is a great idea for checking the anti-inflammatory effectiveness of your diet. Men should aim for a CRP less than 0.55, while women should aim for a CRP less than 1.5.

Foods That Trigger Inflammation

Bad fats

Unfortunately, the standard American diet swings the balance toward excessive amounts of bad prostaglandins. This can increase inflammation and constrict blood vessels, setting the stage for hypertension, heart disease, heart attack, stroke, weight gain, obesity, and diabetes.

While defenders of the dietary status quo poke fun at health advocates or ridicule them as the "food police," the truth is that there are dangers in the types of fats we consume. The main types that trigger inflammation are trans fats, hydrogenated fats, and partially hydrogenated fats. These are generally found in margarines, shortenings, hydrogenated oils, and most baked goods. They are especially prevalent in cake icing, many commercial peanut butters, chips, crackers, cookies, and any foods that list hydrogenated or partially hydrogenated oils on the label. Fried foods—especially those that are deep-fried (e.g., fried chicken, french fries, fried fish)—also increase inflammation.

> **JUST SAY NO**
>
> Aspirin and ibuprofen may seem like quick, easy, and affordable solutions for reducing inflammation. The same is true for various steroids (Prednisone, Cortisone, and Medrol) and nonsteroidal anti-inflammatory drugs. However, keep in mind that when used long term, all of these come with a potentially serious cost, such as the increased likelihood of heart attacks, stroke, and other ailments.

You should also avoid excessive intake of saturated fats, which are found primarily in red meat, pork, processed meats, butter, whole milk, cheese, and poultry skins. All increase your chances of inflammation.

So do omega-6 fats, which are found in vegetable oils, such as safflower, corn, soy, sunflower, and cottonseed oils. Most salad dressings contain these toxic oils. Their labels will usually list "linoleic acid" or "polyunsaturated omega-6."

Corn-fed beef

Corn-fed beef significantly increases inflammation, which is why you should search for "organic" or "grass fed" designations on cuts of steak, hamburger, and other meats. What difference does it make? Grass-fed cattle have approximately six to eight times less fat than grain-fed cattle, as well as two to six times more omega-3 fats. These omega-3s decrease inflammation. This is because the grass the livestock eat typically contains omega-3 fats that are eventually stored in their flesh. Most livestock today are grain fed—usually corn. This increases the omega-6 oils, overall fat, and saturated fats. Both fats are inflammatory, which means that while you enjoy your hamburger or steak, you may be inflaming your body.

By the way, chickens are fed similar to the way livestock are fed. Feeding poultry a grain-based diet causes chickens, as well as their eggs, to be loaded with pro-inflammatory fats.

Sugars and refined carbohydrates

All sugars and refined carbohydrates can fan inflammation in the body. Refined carbohydrates include white bread, white rice, crackers, chips, refined sugary cereals, and potatoes. One study found that overweight women who ate these foods regularly had the highest levels of CRP.[7] Another study at Harvard University discovered that women who ate foods with the highest glycemic load (refined carbohydrates) experienced nearly twice as much inflammation as other women.[8] Women: the more inflammation that exists in your body, the faster you will age and the more wrinkles you will develop. Try keeping that in mind the next time you reach for a soda, dessert, or white bread.

Foods rich in arachidonic acid

Both saturated fats and omega-6 fats can convert to arachidonic acid. Since this acid is a building block for bad prostaglandins, it is wise to limit consumption of this inflammatory fat. Foods rich in arachidonic acid include fatty cuts of red meat and pork, egg yolks, high-fat dairy products, shellfish, and organ meats.

The problem arises especially in men who consume a pound or two of steak, three to four eggs, a pint of ice cream, half a pound of cheese, a few tablespoons of butter, and a quart of whole milk daily. While periodically eating small portions (3 to 6 ounces) of lean, organic red meat is acceptable, eating mammoth-sized steaks or hamburger every day is a recipe for inflammatory disaster. When you eat large amounts of foods rich in arachidonic acid, your body increases its production of enzymes to break down the acid. This produces leukotriene B4 and other inflammatory elements that can cause even more chronic inflammation.

Foods That Control Inflammation

Good fats

Just as bad fats are a source of inflammation, good fats are the best fire extinguishers. Omega-3 fats from cold-water fish, wild fish instead of farm-raised fish, or high-quality omega-3 supplements are the best anti-inflammatory oils. Unfortunately, the standard American diet is low in omega-3 fats and high in the inflammatory omega-6 fats. The recommended ratio of omega-6 fats to omega-3 fats should be four to one. However, most Americans consume these in a ratio closer to twenty to one.

Another good fat that helps decrease inflammation is gamma-linolenic acid, or GLA. Found in borage oil, black currant seed oil, and evening primrose oil, GLA is classified as an omega-6 oil but behaves more like an omega-3. Other good fats include the omega-9 family of fats; among them are olive oil, almonds, avocados, and macadamia nuts. In addition, raw nuts and seeds—such as walnuts, pecans, and flaxseeds—are good anti-inflammatory fats.

Increase fruits and vegetables

With the exception of potatoes and corn, almost all vegetables will help with inflammation. I recommend eating many different vegetables with a diversity of color—and choosing organic. Be aware that some vegetables classified as "nightshades" may trigger inflammation in some individuals, especially those with arthritis. Examples of nightshades are tomatoes, potatoes, peppers, and eggplants. If after eating nightshade vegetables you experience joint aches, swelling, or redness; rashes; or increased arthritis symptoms, you should probably limit or avoid nightshade vegetables. Sometimes the inflammation from eating these vegetables occurs within a day or two. For others, it may occur a few hours after consumption. If you suspect nightshades are causing inflammation, refer to www.worldhealth .net to find a physician experienced in diagnosing and treating food sensitivities.

Some fruits and vegetables are particularly helpful in calming inflammation. Onions, apples, red grapes, and red wine all contain quercetin, a powerful antioxidant that helps quench inflammation. Garlic, ginger, and rosemary sprigs have anti-inflammatory properties. So does curry powder,

FISHY TIP

When shopping for a great source of omega-3 fats to reduce inflammation, keep in mind that all salmon from Alaska is wild, whereas Atlantic salmon is typically farmed. Just because a grocery store or restaurant labels its salmon "wild" doesn't necessarily mean it is. Farmed fish makes up 90 percent of this country's salmon sales, so do your homework to make sure you can trust certain brands, supermarkets, or eating establishments.[9]

WHEN ACTIVITY ITCHES

For most people, food allergy symptoms arrive shortly (if not immediately) after consuming a particular food with allergens. However, for a small segment of the population, such a reaction is conditional on physical activity. Those who have physical-activity-induced food allergies only detect it if they eat a certain food or foods and then work out. As their body temperature increases, symptoms such as itching, light-headedness, hives, asthma, or anaphylaxis can appear. The remedy is as easy as not eating for at least two hours before an activity session.

which contains curcumin, a highly anti-inflammatory spice. In addition, pineapple contains bromelain, an enzyme that decreases inflammation. The herb Boswellia also decreases inflammation. It's best to choose organic produce. (For information on other foods that decrease inflammation, see my book *The Seven Pillars of Health*.)

A sensible program like I recommend succeeds because it includes low-glycemic foods, including plenty of fruits and vegetables. A low-glycemic diet helps users practice portion control, limits bad fats, and encourages the consumption of healthy fats. Essentially, when you learn how to substitute good fats for inflammatory fats; replace high-glygemic, refined carbohydrates with low-glycemic, high-fiber ones; and eat lean, organic, free-range meats in place of high-fat, grain-fed varieties, you dramatically decrease inflammation. Limiting or avoiding sugar, juices, sodas, desserts, and sugary coffees can also help quench these fires.

The Anti-Inflammatory Diet: Taking the Mediterranean Diet to the Next Level

So then, how do you escape this systematic inflammation that is causing so many people so many health problems? First of all, you adopt the Mediterranean diet as the foundation for your day-in, day-out meal planning.

Then, within that framework, balance your pro-inflammatory and anti-inflammatory friendly foods as your body and your CRP tests indicate that you should. This will, of course, initially probably mean adding more anti-inflammatory foods and avoiding the pro-inflammatory ones for a time. I highly recommend Monica Reinagel's *The Inflammation Free Diet Plan* where she presents her years of research to ascribe an Inflammation Free (IF) Rating to the foods we eat. This rating system takes into account more than twenty different factors that contribute to a food's relationship to inflammation. Positive ratings are anti-inflammatory, and foods with negative ratings promote inflammation. Up to a hundred on each scale is considered mildly one way or the other, over a hundred is moderate, and over five hundred is severe.

Looking at her research and adding some of my own, I have organized the following two lists of foods for you to consider adding or subtracting from your diet as your level of systematic inflammation demands.

TOP ANTI-INFLAMMATORY FOODS (ALWAYS CHOOSE ORGANIC WHEN POSSIBLE)	
Fruit	Raspberries, acerola (West Indian) cherries, guava, strawberries, cantaloupe, lemons/limes, rhubarb, kumquat, pink grapefruit, mulberries, blueberries, blackberries
Vegetables	Chili peppers, onions (including scallions and leeks), spinach (greens, including kale, collards, and turnip and mustard greens), sweet potatoes, carrots, garlic
Legumes	Lentils, green beans
Egg Products	Liquid eggs, egg whites
Dairy	Cottage cheese (low fat and nonfat), nonfat cream cheese, plain low-fat Greek yogurt
Fish	Herring, mackerel (not king), wild salmon (not farmed; Alaskan preferred), rainbow trout, sardines, anchovies
Poultry	Goose, duck, free-range organic chicken and turkey
Meat	Pot roast, beef shank, eye of round (beef), flank steak, sirloin tip, prime rib, skirt steak, pork rib chops, pork tenderloin
Cereal	All-Bran, Total, bran flakes, oatmeal, oat bran
Fats/Oils	Safflower oil (high oleic), hazelnut oil, olive oil, avocado oil, almond oil, apricot kernel oil, canola oil, cod liver oil
Nuts/Seeds	Brazil nuts, macadamia nuts, hazelnuts, pecans, almonds, hickory nuts, cashews
Herbs/Spices	Garlic, onion, cayenne, ginger, turmeric, chili peppers, chili powder, curry powder
Sweeteners	Stevia
Beverages	Carrot juice, tomato juice, black or green tea, club soda/seltzer, herbal tea, nonalcoholic wine, spring water

INFLAMMATORY FOODS TO LIMIT OR AVOID	
Fruit	Mango, banana, dried apricots, dried apples, dried dates, canned fruits, raisins
Vegetables	Corn, white potatoes, french fries
Legumes	Baked beans, fava beans (boiled), canned beans
Egg Products	Duck eggs, goose eggs, hard-boiled eggs, egg yolks
Cheeses	Brick cheese, cheddar cheese, Colby cheese, cream cheese (normal and reduced fat)
Dairy	Fruited yogurt, ice cream, butter
Fish	Farmed salmon
Poultry	Turkey (dark meat), Cornish game hen, chicken giblets, chicken liver
Meat	Bacon, veal loin, veal kidney, beef lung, beef kidney, beef heart, beef brain, pork chitterlings, lamb rib chops, turkey breast with skin, turkey wing with skin, all processed meats
Breads	Hot dog/hamburger buns, English muffins, kaiser rolls, bagels, French bread, Vienna bread, blueberry muffins, oat bran muffins
Cereal	Grape-Nuts, Crispix, Corn Chex, Just Right, Rice Chex, corn flakes, Rise Krispies, Raisin Bran, shredded wheat
Pasta/Grain	White rice, brown rice, millet, corn pasta, cornmeal, lasagna noodles, macaroni elbows, regular pasta
Fats/Oils	Margarine, wheat germ oil, sunflower oil, poppy seed oil, grape seed oil, safflower oil, cottonseed oil, palm kernel oil, coconut oil, corn oil
Nuts/Seeds	Poppy seeds, walnuts, pine nuts, sunflower seeds
Sweeteners	Honey, brown sugar, white sugar, corn syrup, powdered sugar
Crackers/ Chips/Cookies	Corn chips, pretzels, graham crackers, saltines, vanilla wafers

INFLAMMATORY FOODS TO LIMIT OR AVOID (continued)	
Desserts	Sweetened-condensed milk, angel food cake, chocolate and vanilla cake with frosting, chocolate chips, heavy whipping cream, ice cream, fruit leather snacks
Candy	Chocolate Kisses, jelly beans, Twix, Almond Joy, milk chocolate bars, Snickers
Beverages	Milk, Gatorade, pineapple juice, orange juice, cranberry juice, lemonade, sodas, sugar-laden soft drinks

These are not complete lists by any means—just some of the more likely "suspects" to watch out for or some of the more helpful helpers to work into your diet. As you read these now, some of these will jump out at you as things you like and need, but you don't have as much of them in your diet as you probably should. Or maybe they are the foods that you know it is time to change your habits about and say good-bye to. The thing to remember is that you have a choice about what you put in your mouth, and now that you have a little more knowledge about these foods, you can begin making healthier diet choices concerning them.

Food Allergies and Sensitivities

Food allergies are a typical inflammatory response often found on the pathway to obesity and diabetes. The most common food allergies are caused by eggs, cow's milk and other dairy products, peanuts, wheat (gluten), soy, tree nuts (such as almonds, cashews, pecans, or walnuts), fish, shellfish, and seeds (sesame and sunflower seeds). An estimated forty to fifty million Americans have environmental allergies, but only about 4 percent of all adults are allergic to foods or food additives. Among children under the age of four, this increases to 7 percent.[10]

Symptoms of food allergies include hives, eczema, rashes, nausea, vomiting, diarrhea, swollen lips, tingling lips or tongue, stomach cramps, asthma, breathing problems, wheezing, anaphylaxis, and sneezing or a runny, stuffy, or itchy nose. These symptoms usually occur within minutes to a few hours after eating the offending food. Food allergies cause significant inflammation; these substances need to be identified and removed from the diet.

Delayed food sensitivities

Another type of allergy poses significant problems for people trying to manage their weight and blood sugar levels. I have observed that many of my obese patients have delayed food sensitivities. The American Allergy and

Immunology Association only allows immunoglobulin E (IgE) reactions to be called "allergy reactions." IgE food allergies produce such symptoms as tingling lips or tongue, swollen lips, or wheezing, generally within minutes to a few hours after eating a food. However, there are three other common, overlooked allergy pathways. Type II, III, and IV are delayed food reactions where symptoms may not occur for hours or even days after ingesting the food. Although these delayed allergy reactions are common, because it usually takes awhile for symptoms to occur, patients and physicians often don't recognize them as such.

Many cases of obesity and weight gain in which no diet works stem from delayed food sensitivities. Other diseases commonly associated with delayed sensitivities include migraine headaches, psoriasis, irritable bowel syndrome, eczema, arthritis, chronic fatigue syndrome, ADD and ADHD, asthma, fibromyalgia, chronic sinusitis, colitis, Crohn's disease, acid reflux, autism, and rosacea. (For information about delayed food sensitivity testing, see Appendix B.)

Increased Intestinal Permeability or Leaky Gut

Delayed food sensitivities usually start in the intestinal tract when the lining of the GI tract becomes inflamed and hyper-permeable. Some doctors term this increased permeability of the intestinal tract "leaky gut." This simply means that the GI tract has become inflamed. Among the many causes are intestinal infections (food poisoning or bacterial, parasitic, viral, or yeast infections), certain medications (aspirin, anti-inflammatory medications, or antibiotics), or ingesting gut-irritating foods and beverages, such as alcohol or hot spices.

An inflamed gut causes the tight junctions between mucosa cells in the small intestines to open. This allows an increased absorption of partially digested proteins. Under normal circumstances the GI tract only absorbs amino acids (not proteins), glucose, and short-chain fatty acids.

However, with increased intestinal permeability, the body absorbs large food proteins, antigens, and toxins. The body then may produce antibodies against harmless foods that we once enjoyed. Since the body now views these foods as invaders, it forms antibodies to fight them. When IgE antibodies and immune complexes form, they may inflame and damage many different tissues and organs. This eventually leads to the diseases I mentioned above, as well as the inability to lose weight. The most common delayed food sensitivities are to dairy, gluten, eggs, peanuts, corn, soy, fish, shellfish, and tree nuts.

Altered GI Flora or Dysbiosis

Although many bacteria are beneficial, some are potentially pathogenic, meaning they are capable of causing disease. Others are full-fledged pathogens. Pathogenic bacteria often make toxins that can be absorbed back into the bloodstream. Bacterial enzymes can also convert bile into chemicals that promote the development of cancer.

The problem for most people is that because doctors are quick to pull the trigger on prescribing antibiotics, these patients' natural beneficial bacteria levels become imbalanced. When patients use antibiotics too often or for too long, it can create an overabundance of pathogenic bacteria. These upset the natural balance in the large intestine by killing off many beneficial bacteria. This can allow more pathogenic bacteria to grow without restraint. Under normal circumstances, massive amounts of bacteria coexist with significantly smaller colonies of yeast. The excessive number of beneficial bacteria prevents these yeasts from enlarging their territory. However, frequent or prolonged use of antibiotics destroys much of the bacteria and does no harm to the yeast, allowing them to grow unchecked. This can lead to chronic inflammation of the GI tract, food cravings, certain food sensitivities, and weight gain.

Unfortunately, when physicians do not recognize this altered gut ecology, they treat the symptoms while ignoring the root issue. They rarely prescribe beneficial bacteria after taking antibiotics and usually do not limit the patient's sugar intake or consumption of fermented and moldy foods. Yet when patients follow through with these easy steps for just a few months, the problem is usually corrected.

Obviously, treating altered GI ecology is more involved than simply popping a few pills. I incorporated ways to restore the GI tract in my books *Dr. Colbert's "I Can Do This" Diet* and *The Bible Cure for Candida and Yeast Infections*. If this is more problematic for you, I urge you to start replenishing your GI tract with beneficial bacteria through a probiotic (beneficial bacteria). Some of the supplements that can help with this are in Appendix B. I would also advise you to avoid all sugar and refined foods for at least three months. In my opinion, altered gut ecology is yet another common cause of obesity, setting the stage for diabetes, that often goes unrecognized by traditional medicine.

Chapter 7

HIDDEN CONTRIBUTOR #4: HORMONE IMBALANCE

Ever closed your eyes and dreamed you were wafting along on a cloud in the sky as you basked in the lilting sounds of Ludwig van Beethoven's *Symphony No. 5*, Dmitri Shostakovich's *Leningrad Symphony*, or Franz Schubert's *Symphony No. 4*? There is something mesmerizing about hearing and watching one hundred masterful musicians weaving their instruments' sounds into a beautiful, sonic tapestry. Yet without one person—the conductor—that tapestry would fray into a cacophonous tattered mat, like a musical version of anarchy.

The conductor leads each individual musician and orchestral section as he or she directs them when to play, how loudly or how softly to play, and essentially what to play, all the while keeping the entire group in synchronized time. Imagine a performance in which every instrument of an orchestra played every note of the score with no regard for volume, tempo, or tone. It would probably sound more like an inexperienced seventh-grade band on the first day of school than an assembly of professional musicians.

The body's hormones are arrayed much like an orchestra's instruments. Each offers something unique and shares a distinct part in bettering the body as a whole. And each needs a conductor. When it comes to hormones, this role is filled by two parts of the brain: the hypothalamus and the pituitary. These two glands are maestros at controlling and manipulating the output of hormones from specific glands.

Over the course of a lifetime, conducting this hormonal orchestra isn't a simple job. In the teen years, it is a cakewalk: hormones such as testosterone from the testes (males), progesterone and estrogen from the ovaries (females), and growth hormones are released in abundant supply. They make beautiful, harmonious music. Our peak hormonal function usually occurs in our late teens and early twenties. This explains why we have such tremendous energy during those years, working all day *and* staying out all night without missing a step. We were in hormonal heaven.

However, as we age—especially after thirty-five—hormonal levels start to sputter. The beautiful hormonal melody misses a few notes and gets off-key once in a while. After the half-century mark, things get worse. The music begins to sound a bit irritating. Sadly, after a dramatic drop in hormonal output for those past sixty, the sounds degenerate from music into just plain noise.

The most tragic thing I find isn't that those in the sixty-and-up crowd are making lousy hormonal music. It's the fact that most physicians miss it by explaining that your potbelly, sagging muscles, high cholesterol, hypertension, depression, and heart disease are all simply signs of aging—so deal with it. No, no, no! These deteriorations are all signs of a dramatic and prolonged drop in key hormones. Your orchestra has been out of tune for so long it has grown accustomed to sour notes. In terms of weight loss, that means you get stuck in obesity.

However, you can turn that around. When properly conducted, your hormones can still play—regardless of age—a key role in losing weight and keeping it off. I will start with a look at the challenges facing women and offer some solutions.

Menopause and Weight Gain

Menopause is defined as having no menstrual cycle for twelve months. It generally occurs around age fifty, but it can begin as early as thirty-five to forty years of age or as late as fifty-five to sixty. Most women spend about a third of their lives in menopause or postmenopause, during which their hormone levels are low. During menopause the ovaries typically stop producing estrogen and progesterone.

STILL GOING…

Even during and after menopause, women can still have elevated estrogen levels. When the ovaries stop producing estrogen, the hormone primarily comes from fat cells, which are able to manufacture estrogen, albeit usually at a lower rate.

Common symptoms include hot flashes, night sweats, vaginal dryness, mood swings, irritability, hair loss, palpitations, lapses in memory, and weight gain. Menopause is also associated with an increased risk of heart disease, osteoporosis, obesity, memory loss, and insulin resistance. During this time women often develop a "menopot," or potbelly. Because of low or fluctuating hormone levels, many menopausal women also experience various severe food cravings. Similar to the cravings some women experience during pregnancy, these strong desires generally revolve around starches such as breads, pasta, and sweets—especially chocolate.

As you can imagine, because of these cravings many women end up overweight or obese during their menopausal years. Depression also runs higher, yet unfortunately most physicians' response is to prescribe an antidepressant. This only complicates the matter and typically leaves patients gaining even more weight. The truth is, most menopausal women simply need a bioidentical estrogen and progesterone found in a transdermal cream. Unfortunately, even taking estrogen in pill or capsule form can cause weight gain and further increase cravings for carbohydrates. That is why I prescribe hormone replacement therapy in transdermal creams or recommend hormone pellet therapy.

Estrogen and Estrogen Dominance

The two hormones needing replenishment during menopause are estrogen and progesterone. I will start by reviewing estrogen, a valuable hormone with more than four hundred vital functions, some of which improve sleep, maintain muscle, increase the metabolic rate, and help to balance neurotransmitters in the brain (which helps reduce food cravings). Estrogen also improves insulin sensitivity, which helps patients struggling with insulin resistance. The bottom line: the correct amount of bioidentical estrogen helps with weight loss in multiple ways. On the flip side, women who lack this vital hormone are more prone to developing serotonin deficiency—which not only causes cravings for sugars and starches but also quickly leads to obesity, leading the way to type 2 diabetes.

The tricky part is that both extremes of estrogen levels can lead down this road. Although low estrogen can cause weight

THE HORMONE CONTROVERSY

For many women, the word *estrogen* took on a new meaning in 2002. That's when a study of more than 160,000 women had to be discontinued after two separate groups receiving treatments of estrogen and an estrogen-progestin combination showed an increase in risk of heart attacks, breast cancer, and stroke. While almost 70 percent of women stopped using hormone replacement therapy entirely, millions of women were left in low-hormone limbo.[1] The truth is, women need not fear natural estrogens. Under a qualified physician's treatment, small doses of bioidentical hormones in the correct ratios as a transdermal cream should be able to control most of the symptoms of menopause and help to program a woman's body for weight loss.

gain, so can having too much. This can especially lead to extra pounds in the abdomen, hips, thighs, and waist. Unfortunately, there are several more severe symptoms associated with excess estrogen. Having excess estrogen levels is known as estrogen dominance, a term coined by the late Dr. John R. Lee. Symptoms include heavy menstrual periods, fluid retention, swollen breasts, fibrocystic breast disease, polycystic ovaries, uterine fibroids, endometriosis, abdominal bloating, mood swings, irritability, depression, anxiety, and an increased risk of breast and uterine cancer.

Estrogen dominance may be caused by taking birth control pills or by synthetic hormone replacement therapy, which involves synthetic hormones that do not function the same as bioidentical ones. Estrogen dominance can also be caused by constipation, impaired elimination of estrogen, obesity, or an increased intake of xenoestrogens. Xenoestrogens are synthetic forms of estrogens found in pesticides, herbicides, petrochemicals, and plastics that are much more powerful than estrogen. Most of our grains and produce are sprayed with pesticides. Similar pesticides are found in meats, especially in the fatty portions.

Remember, most commercial meats come from animals crowded into feedlots where they are fed antibiotics. Their feed is typically treated with insecticides and herbicides. Most of these toxins eventually accumulate in the animals' tissues, especially the fatty tissues, which are then passed on to the consumer. As we consume these passed-along but still powerful xenoestrogens, we are simultaneously creating excess estrogen and programming ourselves for weight gain. Estradiol, for example, is the strongest form of estrogen in the body, yet synthetic estrogens are about two hundred times as potent as estradiol and act as fat magnets. (This is yet another reason why it is so important to purchase organic foods and lean free-range, range-fed, or organic meats.)

If you have estrogen dominance or any of the conditions associated with estrogen dominance that I listed earlier, it is important that you lose weight and take extra-soluble fiber (such as flaxseeds ground up in a coffee grinder) to bind the estrogens and eliminate them. I strongly urge you to switch to organic foods or free-range products with minimal animal fats, and organic skim milk dairy products. Be sure to consume cruciferous vegetables, such as broccoli, cabbage, cauliflower, and brussels sprouts, and take a broccoli supplement such as DIM or indole-3-carbinol. (See Appendix B.) These vegetables help the liver detoxify these hormones and eliminate them from the body.

Progesterone

The second crucial hormone that declines during menopause is progesterone. In fact, both menopausal and postmenopausal women usually have significantly less progesterone than estrogen. Natural progesterone has a calming effect on the body, helps to improve sleep, and acts like a natural antidepressant. However, instead of using this natural progesterone, most physicians give their patients synthetic progesterone, which does not act as a natural antidepressant and also causes weight gain, swelling, acne, edema, an increased risk of blood clots, and other physical problems. These doctors are also quick to prescribe antidepressants for premenopausal and menopausal women, when natural hormone replacement is often all they need.

Decreased progesterone is associated with many symptoms, including mood swings, palpitations, insomnia, irritability, PMS, anxiety, depression, hair loss, decreased sex drive, and weight gain. Because there is such a wide range of symptoms and because many are so common, many gynecologists or family physicians now routinely treat patients exhibiting such symptoms with an antidepressant. For instance, if a woman is experiencing irregular menstrual cycles, severe cramping, or excessive bleeding, it is normal for a doctor to prescribe synthetic progesterone or a birth control pill. Once again, however, *all* of these temporary solutions cause weight gain, which obviously complicates the problem.

In particular, synthetic progestins often increase the appetite and cause weight gain, bloating, fluid retention, acne, and hair loss—almost all the opposite effects of natural progesterone. To avoid this, I prescribe bioidentical progesterone as a transdermal cream, or one to be taken orally for patients with progesterone deficiency. As with estrogen, these hormones are like instruments in an orchestra. They must be balanced, or else they will produce disharmony. Too much progesterone or estrogen can cause weight gain, as can a deficiency in either. If you have numerous symptoms of low progesterone, ask your doctor about taking a salivary hormone test or a blood test for progesterone. See Appendix B to find a doctor who prescribes bioidentical hormones.

SLEEP SOUNDLY

Women with low progesterone levels who suffer from insomnia usually benefit significantly from bioidentical progesterone taken orally at bedtime.

PERIMENOPAUSE

Hormone levels typically begin to change in women in their midthirties, when many women enter perimenopause, the period leading up to menopause that may include some of its symptoms. During perimenopause, women usually start experiencing hormone imbalance with irregular menstrual cycles, cramping, bleeding problems, headaches, breast tenderness, and so forth. In addition, estrogen levels often decline gradually, while progesterone levels usually decline more rapidly. They may even plummet, especially if you are chronically stressed.

Testosterone and Women

Believing that testosterone is unimportant for women, most physicians have followed the idea that women only need to concentrate on estrogen and progesterone levels. However, we now know that testosterone is just as crucial for women for controlling weight, since this powerful hormone helps them to increase muscle mass and strength and to tone muscles. Testosterone also increases sex drive and physical stamina, and it helps with overall weight loss.

Women often start gaining body fat ten years before experiencing menopause, yet most doctors do not even realize that declining testosterone levels usually play a role in this perimenopausal weight gain. As a result, few physicians use testosterone replacement therapy in women. The truth is, women also produce testosterone, and although it amounts to only about a tenth of the male level, it still plays a significant role in keeping pounds off.

Testosterone is produced in a woman's ovaries and adrenal glands. As she ages, her ovaries produce less testosterone, so that with menopause, most of the testosterone is manufactured by the adrenal glands. If her testosterone levels are low or borderline, and she is experiencing the symptoms of low testosterone, I use low doses of testosterone cream or sublingual testosterone tablets. However, obese women who have excessive belly fat may have elevated testosterone levels. Belly fat can raise estrogen levels in men and also may raise testosterone levels in women.

Grumpy Old Man Syndrome

Several years ago a patient I'll call Dan came to see me as a last resort. Fifty-five years old and obese, he had been to numerous physicians for his weight problem and irritability during the previous five years. Initially physicians diagnosed him with mild depression and placed him on Prozac. That did not help, so they switched him to a different antidepressant. After this failed to work, one referred him to a psychiatrist, who promptly placed him on other antidepressants. Of course, these did not help, instead causing him to gain even more weight. Finally he stopped taking any medications and quit going to his psychiatrist and any other physicians.

With no other diseases associated with his obesity, Dan was understandably frustrated with his weight gain, irritability, and his doctors' inability to even remotely help him. And, with no solution in sight, he became increasingly irritable, negative, pessimistic, and angry. He was never prone to these characteristics before age fifty, yet he saw himself turning into the prototypical "grumpy old man." After a friend told him about me, he scheduled an appointment.

While taking Dan's history during his physical, I noticed he had lost a significant amount of pubic and axillary (armpits) hair. I asked him about his sex drive, and he said it had been nonexistent for the past five years. He also hadn't experienced any spontaneous morning erections during that time. In addition, I saw that even though Dan had a potbelly, he had lost significant muscle mass in his arms and legs and had replaced much of that muscle with fat.

These symptoms made it evident that he was suffering from hypogonadism, or low testosterone levels. Another name for this is andropause, or male menopause; some even label it "grumpy old man syndrome." Essentially, Dan's testosterone levels were extremely low. As Dan showed, general symptoms of low testosterone in men include a decrease in any or all of the following: sex drive, spontaneous early morning erections, mental acuity, competitiveness, muscle mass and tone, strength, and stamina. Along with these symptoms, men suffering from hypogonadism often experience grumpiness, irritability, anger, depression, loss of pubic and axillary hair, fatigue, and an overall feeling of burnout.

While hypogonadism only affects approximately four million men in the United States,[2] researchers have found that more than a third of all men age forty-five and older have low testosterone levels.[3] Among this age group, obesity, diabetes, and high blood pressure all affect testosterone levels. A recent study of more than 2,100 men age forty-five and older found that those with obesity were 2.4 times more likely as other men the same age to have hypogonadism. Those with type 2 diabetes were 2.1 times more likely to have low testosterone levels, and those with hypertension were 1.8 times more likely to have low testosterone. In addition, men with elevated cholesterol, prostate disease, and asthma have increased chances of hypogonadism.[4]

Unfortunately, most doctors overlook low testosterone levels and usually attribute these diseases to aging. As men age, their testosterone levels typically drop by about 1 percent each year, starting at age forty. Yet another recent study indicates that the difference in declining testosterone among obese men, compared to non-obese men ages forty to seventy, is equivalent to adding ten years of age.[5] In other words, hypogonadism speeds up the aging process, largely because of its link to weight gain. Researchers from the University of California–San Diego School of Medicine found that men with low testosterone levels were three times more likely to suffer from metabolic syndrome than men with higher testosterone.[6] As I discussed previously, metabolic syndrome is closely associated with obesity.

If you have some of the symptoms listed in this section, ask your physician about getting a blood test to check testosterone levels. I also recommend nutritional supplements to prevent prostate problems and to prevent the testosterone from converting to estrogen. The treatment in each of these cases is hormone replacement. A medical doctor experienced in transdermal natural hormone replacement therapy or hormone pellet therapy should do this. For more information on finding such a physician, visit www.worldhealth.net.

Dan's Remedy

After placing Dan on a testosterone cream and adjusting the dose until his testosterone levels returned to normal, Dan's symptoms faded away. Five years of frustration were over within a few months. Because of his obesity, I also put Dan on a low-glycemic program with an aerobic exercise and strengthening program. His transformation proved remarkable. Dan lost his grumpiness, irritability, and pessimism; he became energetic and happy and regained his competitive edge. His sex drive returned, along with his pubic and axillary hair. He gained muscle mass and burned off most of his belly fat. His waist measurement dropped from 45 inches to 37 inches in just eight months.

Growth Hormone

The last hormone in the body orchestra I would like to review is growth hormone. Serving a variety of purposes, this hormone is most evident as we grow taller

MUCH ADO ABOUT NOTHING?

Amidst all the hype in recent years surrounding athletes taking banned growth hormones, a recent study proves the drug actually may not be doing much to improve athletic performance. Compiling information from more than two dozen studies since 1966, Stanford University researchers discovered that although growth hormone correlated with leaner body mass (which usually means more muscle), that didn't necessarily translate to being faster, quicker, or stronger. In fact, a few studies proved the hormone generated more lactate—which, as a by-product of exercise, caused increased muscle fatigue. However, it should be noted that Stanford researchers used low levels of growth hormone in their testing, while various athletes may be using much larger dosages that generate "stronger" results (and, presumably, just as potent side effects).[7]

in childhood and adolescence. It stimulates both growth and cell reproduction, increases muscle mass, reduces body fat, helps control insulin and sugar levels, and assists in retaining calcium throughout the body. It assists with many other functions as well. Therefore, when we lack growth hormone, our growth—as you would expect by its name—levels off. In general, the older we get, the less growth hormone we produce. Symptoms of low growth hormone include thin lips, droopy eyelids, sagging cheeks, loose skin folds under the chin, thin muscles, floppy triceps, a fat droopy abdomen, sagging back muscles, thin skin, and thin soles of the feet—all typical signs of aging.

In 1990, a study directed by Dr. Daniel Rudman unveiled a potential remedy for this. As published in the *New England Journal of Medicine*, Rudman and his colleagues at the Medical College of Wisconsin gave twelve men injections of human growth hormone (HGH), a hormone produced by the pituitary gland in the brain. The body's production of HGH naturally declines with age, which is why Rudman's study became particularly interesting to the medical world. Though Rudman only tested a dozen men, they were between sixty-one and eighty-one, with bodies varying from frail to flabby to obese. Each recipient receiving HGH seemingly turned back the clock decades, growing stronger, leaner, and more energetic. Meanwhile, those in the control group who did not receive HGH revealed no significant change in lean body mass or fatty tissue.[8]

Rudman later followed up on his study by injecting twenty-six different elderly men with HGH. This time he discovered the recipients not only gained muscle tone they had years earlier in their youth, but they also regrew livers and spleens, along with other tissue.[9]

Despite seemingly representing a fountain of youth, HGH does have side effects, including acromegaly, which is overgrowth of the skeleton and organs. In addition, some HGH users have experienced insulin resistance, paresthesias, elevated blood sugar, joint aches, water retention, and carpal tunnel syndrome. Many experts fear that HGH may increase the risk of cancer.

However, you do not have to take injections of HGH to increase your growth hormone. Balancing other hormones also helps raise growth hormone levels. In males, it is important to normalize testosterone levels; in females, the key balance is between estrogen, progesterone, testosterone, and thyroid. In addition, supplementing with melatonin at bedtime, DHEA, and pregnenolone, and getting adequate sleep can help raise growth hormone levels.

I have found that when I balance other hormones in my patients, supplement them with melatonin, DHEA, and pregnenolone, and ensure that they get adequate sleep, they generally do not need growth hormone. For adults who are in the feeble and flabby categories, though, growth hormone injections may not be out of the question if they have true adult growth hormone deficiency.

We have looked at four of the major players in the hormonal orchestra. When conducted properly, these hormones can play a key role in helping you burn fat and build muscle. In combination with proper nutrition and exercise, they create harmonious music—the way the body intended.

In section II I will review the role food plays in reversing diabetes.

Section II

HOW FOOD PLAYS A PART

Chapter 8

HOW METABOLISM WORKS

Whether a nightly weather report showing the day's cloudscape or a montage of a busy street corner's ebb and flow of people, I love watching time-lapse videos. Observing hours, days, weeks, or months of time condensed into mere seconds fascinates me—and apparently it captivates others as well. Photographer John Novotny says that time-lapse photography has a way of affecting people intuitively: "They react to it with wonder, as if the act of making it surreal makes it more real, more beautiful. Of course, you can never beat the real thing, but...if done correctly, you can capture the essence of a place and portray it in a different way."[1]

My interest in this unique form originated with a documentary I saw years ago. It used time-lapse filming to capture the effects of the ocean on the coastline. I sat mesmerized as I watched waves pound away at the rocks, day after day, as tides flowed in and out. At first glance it appeared the water had no particular effect. Even after several years the coast essentially looked the same. Yet the producers proved that had their video been able to track thousands of years, I would have seen an entirely different landscape formed. By repeatedly and ceaselessly beating down the shoreline, the ocean actually wore down the rocks. Eventually the power of gradual erosion can reshape seemingly immovable structures.

In the same way that oceans can eat away at the shoreline, repeat dieting—what many refer to as yo-yo dieting—has a similar effect on our bodies. The damage it causes wears down our metabolism. Generally, yo-yo diets decrease muscle mass and increase body fat. Even without dieting, after age thirty-five the average person loses between five and seven pounds of muscle mass every ten years.[2] However, repeat dieters lose even more muscle mass. Even with many diets that result in weight loss, only approximately half of the pounds you lose are fat. The remainder is usually metabolically active muscle and water.

I cannot overemphasize how detrimental this is to gaining sustained control over your weight. Muscle is extremely valuable! Muscle cells burn about seventy times more calories than fat cells, which is why they are so crucial for maintaining weight loss.

Unfortunately, each time you hop on and off another diet, you typically lose valuable muscle and regain extra fat. Even worse, you gradually become fatter by dramatically lowering your metabolic rate. Studies show that with every decade of muscle loss, your metabolism also decreases by about 5 percent.[3] In essence, every time you drop another attempt at dieting, the more difficult you make the next one.

Before explaining how to halt this cycle and restore your metabolic system, we need to first look at how metabolism works.

Burn While You Rest

Metabolism is defined as the chemical processes continuously occurring in living cells or organisms that are essential for the maintenance of life.[4] It is the sum total of all chemical reactions in the body. Keep in mind that your tissues and organs never take a break. Your heart always pumps, your lungs always draw in breaths, and your liver never stops with its five hundred different functions, such as filtering the blood; removing toxins; processing fats, proteins, and carbohydrates; producing bile; and detoxifying chemicals, toxins, and metabolic waste. Your brain and nervous system, digestive system, immune system, hormones, bones, joints, muscles, and every tissue of your body all require energy.

These functions all contribute to your metabolic rate. Since it takes energy for your heart to beat, your lungs to breathe, and your organs to function properly, the metabolic rate is simply the rate at which you burn calories in a non-active state. When considered over a twenty-four-hour period, this is called the basal metabolic rate (BMR), or resting metabolic rate. You typically burn about 75 percent of your calories during a state of rest. As I will discuss later, several things influence your metabolic rate, including stress level, muscle mass, eating behaviors, food choices, and activity level.

One of the biggest factors that affect the metabolic rate is skipping meals, which I've already mentioned. When you do not eat for more than twelve hours, your metabolic rate goes down by about 40 percent. This sets you up for weight gain, which is compounded by consuming high-carbohydrate, high-fat foods, since your body will not burn as many calories in this lowered metabolic state. This is also why eating a healthy breakfast (literally breaking a "fast" through the night) is so essential. Individuals who eat breakfast are typically leaner than those who skip breakfast because this meal helps increase their metabolic rate.

As you might guess, body fat is not a metabolically active tissue. Muscle tissue, on the other hand, is extremely metabolically active. The more muscle you have, the higher your metabolic rate. The more fat, the slower your metabolic rate. Put another way: it takes far more energy to maintain a pound of muscle than a pound of fat. A good way to increase your metabolic rate is to increase your muscle mass and decrease your body fat.

All in the Calculations

Figuring out a ballpark BMR is easy.* There are more specific formulas for calculating your BMR, but to keep our discussion simple, I will share a general formula. There are three easy steps: First, simply multiply your weight in pounds by ten. Second, determine the number of calories you burn in a day by multiplying the number of minutes you exercise each day by four. Third, add this total to the first number.

For example, if you weigh 200 pounds and exercise thirty minutes a day, you would calculate your calories burned per day as follows:

- Body weight in pounds times ten (200 pounds x 10 = 2,000)
- Number of minutes exercised times four (30 minutes x 4 = 120)
- Add 2,000 to 120 = 2,120 calories burned per day

Remember that this is only a rough estimate of the metabolic rate; it does not apply to people who are metabolically compromised or have a depressed metabolic rate. Please refer to *Dr. Colbert's "I Can Do This" Diet* for more scientific formulas for BMR.

Easier Said Than Done

How many times have you heard someone make the simplistic statement, "Losing weight isn't rocket science. All it takes is eating less and exercising more." Many of my obese patients would like to wring the necks of all the well-meaning but insensitive people who offer this as word of "advice." As if these patients never tried that!

When it comes to weight loss, it is true that to shed pounds, we usually need to eat less and exercise more. However, what happens when doing these things doesn't work? What do you do when you have followed every diet and exercise program to the tee and still haven't seen results?

If this describes you, first let me remind you that you are not alone. As

---

* When calculating BMR, it's important to realize that the typical male has significantly more muscle mass than a typical female, while women usually have a significantly higher amount of body fat than men. Therefore a one-size-fits-all BMR is not entirely accurate or realistic. The formula I discuss here is a very crude way to measure your BMR.

we explore the various reasons why people get stuck in their efforts to lose weight, you will see that many of these factors are reaching epidemic proportions. If you suffer from one or more of them, you are in the company of millions—and the club is growing. Second, know that you may be metabolically compromised. All that means is that your metabolism is sluggish. Somehow—usually through chronic weight-loss diets and binge eating—it has become impaired to the point of barely working. This means your body isn't burning fuel the way it should be.

BREATHING TEST: THE BEST WAY TO MEASURE YOUR BMR

A routine pulmonary lab test, called indirect calorimetry, can measure oxygen consumption, carbon dioxide production, and respiratory exchange rate. This provides accurate and useful information in providing a detailed picture of the body's metabolic processes at rest.[5]

This can happen for a myriad of reasons, several of which you can find at www.thecandodiet.com. However, the overall result is that your body gets locked into *storing* fat instead of *burning* it. Sadly, many obese and metabolically compromised Americans are unaware of the factors that have contributed to their condition. With that in mind, let's examine some of the major factors that can severely affect metabolic rate.

Chronic Stress Lowers Metabolic Rate

As I explained in chapter 4, chronic stress lowers the metabolic rate. Our bodies are designed to secrete two stress hormones when we are stressed: epinephrine and cortisol. A "fight-or-flight" hormone, epinephrine works immediately by racing through our bodies when triggered by such stressors as an emergency, running late for an appointment, or an argument with a spouse. When our bodies are unable to fight or flee, we become like rush-hour commuters stuck in bumper-to-bumper traffic on the interstate—we are left literally stewing in our own stress juices. Epinephrine revs up the stress response by raising our blood pressure and increasing both our heart rate and our breathing. When the perceived stress is over, the epinephrine level typically drops back to normal.

On the other hand, cortisol works more slowly, giving us stamina to cope with long-term stress. However, when the stress response becomes stuck as a result of long-term stress, the ongoing elevation of cortisol causes the body to continually release sugar into the bloodstream from glycogen. Glycogen is simply stored sugar, generally held in the liver and muscles. When glycogen is released into the bloodstream, it causes insulin levels to rise, which in turn lowers the blood sugar. Low blood sugar causes more cortisol to be released, leading to weight gain. Excessive insulin also causes the body to store fat in adipose tissue, while also preventing the body from releasing fat from the tissues, even during exercise. In other words, stress programs us for fat storage and contributes significantly to insulin resistance.

Elevated cortisol levels can also cause the body to burn muscle tissue as fuel. Cortisol is a catabolic hormone, which means it causes the body to break down muscle to produce energy, leading to an even lower metabolic rate. As any weightlifter knows, muscle tissue is pricey fuel; we sacrifice our metabolic rate when we burn muscle tissue as fuel. Cortisol is the only hormone that increases as we age.

Certain foods and beverages will raise cortisol levels, including everyday items such as caffeinated beverages and coffee. In fact, drinking two cups of coffee raises your cortisol levels by approximately 30 percent within a single hour. I am not recommending that you stop drinking coffee, since it does have health benefits. However, I recommend a maximum of two cups a day.

Eating excessive amounts of sugar, white bread, and other high-glycemic foods without the proper ratio of protein, fats, and fiber can cause hypoglycemic episodes. These are bouts with low blood sugar that also raise cortisol levels. Whenever your blood sugar drops, your body is naturally signaled to increase cortisol production. Another way this can happen is through food allergies and sensitivities and by skipping meals and snack times.

Your Gender Plays a Part

Women typically have a higher percentage of body fat and lower metabolic rate than men. There is currently no consensus on a specific "healthy" range of body fat percentage, and ranges vary according to age. However, most studies indicate a good goal for women is to keep your body fat under 30 percent (for women, obese is defined as a body fat percentage—not BMI—greater than 33 percent; 31–33 percent is borderline). For men, that goal is less than 20 percent (for men, obese is defined as greater than 25 percent; 21–25 percent is borderline).[6] By design, women have a lower metabolic rate than men because they typically carry an additional 7 to 8 percent of fat, even at a healthy weight. Add to this the fact that a woman's metabolic rate declines at the rate of approximately 5 percent per decade of her life, starting at age twenty.

Inactivity and Muscle Loss

With aging, sedentary individuals have a significant loss of muscle mass. Earlier I stated that adults naturally lose 5 to 7 pounds of muscle every ten years after age thirty-five; as you might guess, inactivity further accelerates this process. The less active we are, the more body fat we keep—and, naturally, the more muscle we lose. By age sixty, most people have lost about 28 pounds of muscle and replaced most of that with much more fat.

I have found this to be especially true among women. I check body fat measurements on all my weight-loss patients and have commonly encountered women with 50 percent body fat or more. Yet it is extremely rare to find this among male patients. Most high-body-fat cases stem from a combination of gender and lack of exercise, plus metabolic compromise. Obviously, women have a disadvantage by carrying a higher percentage of body fat; generally, they do not lose weight as fast as men. Because of this, it is even more important to educate them about the effects exercise has on metabolism, as well as help them understand the unique challenges they face. A sedentary lifestyle compounds the situation and increases their chances of obesity, laying a foundation for developing type 2 diabetes.

> **SIT OR GET FIT?**
>
> Obese people sit down an average of 152 minutes more each day than more slender individuals.[7]

Could Your Medication Be to Blame?

A common side effect of certain medications is weight gain. These medications include birth control pills, hormone replacement therapy, prednisone and other steroids, various antidepressants, antipsychotic medications, lithium, insulin and insulin-stimulating medications, cholesterol-lowering medications, some anticonvulsant medications, some antihistamines, and certain blood pressure pills, such as beta blockers. Ironically, many physicians treat diseases caused by obesity such as hypertension, diabetes, depression, and elevated cholesterol with the very medications that lower the metabolic rate and result in more weight gain. That is why I typically use vitamins, supplements, and other nutrients in conjunction with a sensible eating plan to treat obesity-associated problems rather than just medications.

Thyroid Problems Affect Your Metabolic Rate

Though often overlooked in the weight-loss equation, a low or sluggish thyroid can also cause a decreased metabolic rate. I have seen hundreds of cases in which patients reached the end of their rope after adhering to every diet under the sun but never losing weight, only to discover their thyroid was inhibiting their progress. Thyroid blood tests should be checked regularly to ensure that the thyroid is functioning normally.

Although men can develop thyroid disease as well, the overwhelming majority of those suffering from thyroid issues are women. An estimated thirteen million American women have some kind of thyroid dysfunction.[8] The sad part is that many of them do not even know it and struggle with weight loss (along with other issues) their entire lives. I discuss the reasons why I believe this goes undiagnosed in *Dr. Colbert's "I Can Do This" Diet*. Researchers say that about 10 percent of younger women and 20 percent of women over age fifty regularly experience mild thyroid problems that impact their weight, attitude, and overall health.[9]

The two main hormones produced by the thyroid gland are thyroxine (T4) and triiodothyronine (T3). Most of the thyroid hormone in the body, or around 80 percent, is T4. T3 is the active form of thyroid hormone and is several times stronger than T4. It is also very important for weight loss. Eighty percent of the T3 in our bodies comes from the conversion of T4 to T3 in such organs and tissues as the kidneys, liver, and muscle. Both of these thyroid hormones gradually decline with age. Yet many obese people may show signs of a sluggish thyroid. I believe one of the main reasons for this is because some are poor converters of T4 to T3. After seeing hundreds of obese people in my practice struggle to convert T4 to T3, I have identified the following reasons for their poor conversion: chronic unremitting stress, taking certain medications (birth control, estrogen and HRT, beta-blockers, chemotherapy, theophylline, lithium, and Dilantin), eating certain foods (soy, excessive consumption of raw cruciferous vegetables, low-fat diets, low-carb diets, and low-protein diets), and excessive alcohol intake.

Half the Equation

Every overweight individual has a reason for his or her overweight condition. Yet sadly, most who have struggled unsuccessfully with diets over the long haul never discover the underlying reasons for their inability to shed pounds. In this chapter I have touched on many of these various causes as they relate to metabolic rate, ranging from skipping meals to chronic dieting to chronic stress to aging to medications to low thyroid. In doing so, I have tried to help you understand the many ways your metabolic rate can be affected—which you now know directly influences maintaining weight loss and blood sugar levels.

This is only half the equation, however. Revealing how metabolism works is essential for understanding how to lose pounds and keep them off. Just as important is knowing the solution: developing a low-glycemic lifestyle. With that in mind, in the next chapter I will look at how to raise your metabolic rate and keep off those pounds for good.

Chapter 9

THE GLYCEMIC INDEX AND GLYCEMIC LOAD

Thirty-five-year-old Barbara had battled obesity since first giving birth ten years earlier. After her third child's birth, she was carrying around an extra 80 pounds of weight and an equal amount of frustration. Numerous diets had helped her shed 5 or 10 pounds, but after these short-term fixes she always gained the weight back—sometimes more. Sound familiar?

Barbara assumed the main culprit was her hectic schedule. She worked full-time, carpooled children to and from school and other activities, prepared dinner, and cleaned house. This pace left Barbara little time every morning to prepare food for her family, eat, and clean up. So instead of depriving her family, she cut back on her consumption. She usually skipped breakfast, grabbing a cup of coffee (loaded with cream and sugar) on the way out the door and wolfing down a bagel or doughnut at the office. For lunch she ate out—often a hamburger, french fries, and a Diet Coke. Almost every afternoon she wandered into the break room for a snack left by generous coworkers: doughnuts, cookies, bagels, cake, or chips.

After work Barbara prepared dinner for her family, which typically consisted of bread (rolls or biscuits), meat, starch (including potatoes, rice, or pasta), and a vegetable. She assumed she must be doing something right, since her children were at a healthy weight and her husband was not overweight. Still, she struggled to understand her 80-pound surplus when she ate the same dinners as the rest of her family.

Controlling Blood Sugar and Insulin

Unbeknownst to Barbara, she was choosing foods that raised her blood sugar, spiked her insulin levels, and programmed her for weight gain and diabetes. Like most Americans, among her core problems was consuming too many processed carbohydrates. Unfortunately, most of the carbohydrates we eat are highly refined; our bodies rapidly convert them to sugar. Take, for example, white bread. The wheat in white bread is highly processed and refined. During the milling process, the wheat grains are cracked

83

and pulverized by a series of rollers. The starchy endosperm portion of the grain, which is high in carbohydrates, is separated from the bran, which contains much healthier fiber, magnesium, and vitamins. The grains are also separated from the wheat germ, which contains polyunsaturated fats and vitamins. The wheat germ and fiber are sold to health food stores while the general public gets the rest. After processing the starchy endosperm, machines grind it more, bleach it white, and eventually turn it into flour. This flour is used to make bagels, breads, buns, cereals, crackers, cookies, muffins, pasta, pretzels, and cakes. Unfortunately, this commonly used but highly refined flour usually raises the blood sugar and stimulates the release of insulin, setting people up for weight gain.

That is exactly what happened to Barbara. When she paused long enough for breakfast instead of skipping it, she usually drank coffee with sugar and ate a fattening bagel (as bad as a doughnut) at work. The sugar in the coffee and the highly processed carbohydrates in the bagel caused Barbara's blood sugar to rise. Once eaten, processed carbohydrates behave like sugars in the GI tract and are absorbed rapidly, causing a sugar spike in the bloodstream. To lower the blood sugar, the pancreas secretes insulin to drive the sugar into the tissues of the body. However, when we consume sugar or highly processed carbohydrates and fail to complement them with sufficient quantities of proteins, fats, and fiber, this poor fuel mixture often causes too much insulin to be secreted by the pancreas.

Why is weight gain so important? Because your waistline is your lifeline. If it increases, your blood sugar will typically increase; if it decreases, so will your blood sugar. When your blood sugar rises rapidly after consuming sugary foods, refined carbohydrates, and insufficient fiber, you usually feel happy, good, energetic, full, and satisfied. However, if the pancreas secretes excessive amounts of insulin, your blood sugar may come crashing down. This, in turn, can cause you to feel spacey, sweaty, lethargic, sluggish, irritable, hungry, light-headed, jittery, and anxious. In addition, your heart may race or you may develop a headache. Since the brain's hunger center immediately detects when the blood sugar falls, it sends out hunger signals.

Whenever Barbara felt these sugar-related symptoms and hunger pangs,

YOUNG AND SWEET

Sugary-sweet cereals were introduced in the early 1950s, when companies first targeted children in their advertisements. Among the first cereals to debut was Kellogg's aptly named Sugar Smacks, which contained an astounding 56 percent sugar.[1] The company later renamed the product Honey Smacks, but don't let name that fool you; sugar is still the number one ingredient on its label.

she searched for a snack in the break room, grabbing a Snickers bar or a leftover doughnut to make her symptoms go away. Unfortunately, this kick-started the vicious cycle, raising her blood sugar once again. As a result, her body was programmed for weight gain. Getting trapped in this cycle also leads one down the road to diabetes.

For Barbara, the main culprits were skipping meals, high-glycemic snacks, and excessive insulin. This hormone is a double-edged sword; although it is needed for good health, too much insulin sets people up for weight gain, obesity, type 2 diabetes, and a host of deadly diseases. Excessive insulin in the bloodstream is called hyperinsulinemia, and when we elevate our insulin levels, we program our bodies to store fat. If these levels remain elevated for too long, we can develop insulin resistance, in which the body's tissues no longer respond normally to insulin.

When this occurs, insulin sends blood sugar into the muscles and liver to be stored as glycogen, but it also causes fat to accumulate in the liver, in the blood (in the form of elevated triglycerides), in the muscle cells, and especially in the abdomen, causing an ever-expanding waistline. This also prevents the body from releasing stored fat, even with exercise. Elevated insulin levels and insulin resistance are associated with many diseases. Among them are type 2 diabetes, heart disease, hypertension, polycystic ovary syndrome, autoimmune disease, Alzheimer's disease, and even some cancers.

Glycemic Index 101

To get a better feel for how quickly insulin levels shot up in individuals after they consumed carbohydrates, doctors and scientists created the glycemic index. This was first identified in the early 1980s by Drs. David Jenkins and Thomas Wolever, two professors of nutrition at the University of Toronto in Canada. In their studies they focused on individuals with type 2 diabetes and found that certain carbohydrates increased blood sugar levels and insulin levels, while other carbohydrates did not. They followed this up by testing hundreds of different foods to determine their glycemic index value. Because their methods and findings have proven so reliable, they are the standard by which we measure the internal processing of foods.

In essence, the glycemic index gives an indication of the rate at which different carbohydrates and foods break down to release sugar into the bloodstream. More precisely, it assigns a numeric value to how rapidly the blood sugar rises after consuming a food that contains carbohydrates. Keep in mind the glycemic index is only for carbohydrates, not fats or proteins. Sugars and carbohydrates that are digested rapidly, such as white bread, white rice, and instant potatoes, rapidly increase blood sugar. These are high-glycemic foods and have a glycemic index of 70 or higher.

On the other hand, if foods containing carbohydrates are digested slowly and therefore release sugars gradually into the bloodstream, they have a glycemic index value of 55 or lower. These foods include most vegetables and fruits, beans, peas, lentils, sweet potatoes, and the like.

RULE OF THUMB: THE GLYCEMIC INDEX

- Low-glycemic foods: 55 or less
- Medium-glycemic foods: 56 to 69
- High-glycemic foods: 70 or above

In truth, there is nothing fancy about the glycemic index. One of the most important factors that can determine a food's glycemic index value is to what degree the food has been processed. Generally speaking, the more highly processed, the higher its glycemic index value; the more natural a food, the lower its value.

Because these foods cause the blood sugar to rise more slowly, blood sugar levels are stabilized for a longer period of time. Low-glycemic foods also cause satiety hormones to be released in the small intestines, which satisfies you for longer periods of time. As an example of the various glycemic index values for different foods, glucose has a value of 100, while broccoli and cabbage—both of which contain little or no carbohydrates—have a value of 0 to 1.

The Glycemic Load

Almost twenty years after Drs. Jenkins and Wolever came up with their measurement, researchers at Harvard University developed a new way of classifying foods that took into account not only the glycemic index value of a food but also the quantity of carbohydrates that particular food contains. This is called the glycemic load (GL). It serves as a guide as to how much of a particular carbohydrate or food we should eat.

For a while, nutritionists scratched their heads over patients who wanted to lose weight and were eating low-glycemic foods yet weren't shedding many pounds. Some actually gained weight. Through the GL they discovered that over-consuming many low-glycemic foods can actually lead to weight gain. Not surprisingly, many patients were eating as many low-glycemic foods as they wanted, simply because they had been told that foods with a low value promoted weight loss. They needed to know the whole story, which is how the glycemic load balanced the picture.

A food's GL is determined by multiplying the glycemic index value by the quantity of carbohydrates a serving contains (in grams), and then dividing that number by 100. The actual formula looks like this:

- (Glycemic Index Value x Carb Grams Per Serving) ÷ 100 = Glycemic Load

To show you how important the GL is, let me offer some examples. Some wheat pastas have a low glycemic index value, which makes many dieters think they're automatically a key to losing weight. However, if a serving size of that wheat pasta is too large, it may sabotage your weight-loss efforts. Despite a low glycemic index value, the pasta's GL is high. Another example is white potatoes, which have a GL double that of yams. On the other end of the scale, watermelon has a high glycemic index value but a very low GL, which makes it OK to eat in a larger quantity.

Don't worry, though. You will not have to calculate the GL for every item at every meal you eat. Instead, I will teach you a simple method to calculate portion sizes of foods. The main point is that by understanding the GL, you can identify which low-glycemic foods can cause trouble if you eat too much of them. These include low-glycemic breads, low-glycemic rice, sweet potatoes, yams, low-glycemic pasta, low-glycemic cereals, and so forth. As a general rule, any large quantity of a low-glycemic "starchy" food will usually have a high GL.

GLYCEMIC INDEX VALUES OF COMMON FOODS[2]	
Food*	Glycemic Index Value
Asparagus	15
Broccoli	15
Celery	15
Cucumber	15
Green beans	15
Low-fat yogurt (artificially sweetened)	15
Peppers (all varieties)	15
Spinach	15
Zucchini	15
Tomatoes	15
Cherries	22

GLYCEMIC INDEX VALUES OF COMMON FOODS (continued)	
Food*	**Glycemic Index Value**
Green peas	22
Black beans	30
Milk (skim)	32
Apples	36
Spaghetti (whole wheat)	37
All-Bran cereal	42
Lentil soup (canned)	44
Orange juice	52
Bananas	53
Potato (sweet)	54
Rice (brown)	55
Popcorn	55
Muesli	56
Whole-wheat bread	69
Watermelon	72
Doughnut	75
Rice cakes	82
Corn flakes	84
Potato (baked)	85
Baguette (French bread)	95
Parsnips	97
Dates	103

* To look up the glycemic index values of other foods not listed above, go to www.thecandodiet.com.

Keep in mind also that if you use the GL (the glycemic load), you will probably be eating more of an Atkins-type diet with lots of fats and proteins and few carbohydrates. This is not a healthy way to eat and can cause insulin resistance due to excessive consumption of the wrong fats, increasing one's risk of developing prediabetes and diabetes.

Some of the foods with high glycemic index values that you need to limit or avoid are instant potatoes, instant rice, white rice, French bread, white bread, corn, processed oats, most boxed cereals, baked potatoes, mashed potatoes, cooked carrots, honey, raisins, dried fruit, candy bars, crackers, cookies, ice cream, and pastries. If you are diabetic, you should eat these foods rarely or simply avoid them and mainly choose non-starchy carbohydrates such as broccoli, green beans, asparagus, and so on.

Too Good to Be True?

When I first met Barbara, she was ready to throw in the weight-loss towel. Yet within a matter of weeks we discovered the two core issues holding her back: meals and the types of foods she ate. First, Barbara started eating three balanced meals a day, along with a healthy midafternoon snack. Second, she switched from high-glycemic carbs to delicious low-glycemic carbs with a low GL. In her own words, the transformation was "simply amazing." She no longer craved sugars and starches, and she felt satisfied and energetic. Following a sensible eating plan enabled Barbara to lose 80 pounds in less than a year, all without dieting or starving herself.

Depending on your current situation, it is possible to see similar results in the same amount of time. This program incorporates both low glycemic index foods and low glycemic load foods, which is why the information in this chapter is so crucial to understand. Although you don't have to know the details or history behind every glycemic term, it helps to have a basic understanding of the glycemic index and glycemic load—and how they can affect your weight-loss success.

Often people will tell me after being on my low glycemic program for a few months that they find it hard to believe it can be this easy. I don't mean to sugarcoat (pardon my word choice) the journey; it can be tough for those who have to overcome multiple obstacles, such as lifelong habits and hereditary influences. Yet even these people are amazed at my relative lack of restrictions. You must eat the same types of foods to lose weight as you do to maintain weight loss. The only difference is that portion sizes will change. You won't have to deprive yourself. Instead you will eat delicious healthy foods that will significantly reduce hunger cravings and help control your appetite. The key is to make sure you eat modest portions and with the correct fuel mixture of good proteins, good fats, and adequate fiber.

My goals are to emphasize moderation so that people can still enjoy their favorite foods, be able to follow a sensible plan for the rest of their lives, and help prevent or overcome diabetes. (Remember, always check with your doctor before starting any weight-loss or dietary plan.) It is not necessary to starve yourself or subsist on "rabbit food." Eating sensibly means you can have increased energy, better sleep, and improved overall health. You won't have to cook different foods for the rest of your family, either. A sensible program like my Rapid Waist Reduction Diet (chapters 17–19) is healthy for children, the elderly, and patients with diabetes, heart disease, or most other diseases.

I want to help you particularly lose weight in the abdominal area, therefore reducing your waist size. You will also improve your bowel regularity with a high-fiber eating plan. Many patients even say it slows down the aging process; they claim to feel younger.

If all those reasons are not enough to follow a good program, here is another one that should catch your attention: your children will be healthier. I have seen countless families turn their lives around when Mom or Dad start eating better and, for sheer convenience's sake, include everyone else. In every case where a concerted effort included the children, they became healthier and more resistant to disease, and they lost weight if they were overweight or obese. They typically had more energy, were able to concentrate better, and behaved better, which often resulted in better grades at school.

Too good to be true? I don't think so, but you will never know until you make the change. Improved health, longevity, and resistance to disease—especially obesity, prediabetes, and diabetes—for you and your family are the rewards for healthy food choices.

Chapter 10

WHAT ABOUT BREAD AND OTHER CARBS?

Carbs. Americans love them. And we need them. The truth is, certain carbohydrates are critical for good health. When combined with the correct portions of fats and proteins, good carbs give you energy, calm your mood, keep you full and satisfied by turning off hunger, and assist in weight loss. They also help you to enjoy meals and snacks, enable you to handle stress better, allow you to sleep more soundly, improve your bowel functions, and give you an overall feeling of well-being.

However, as with so many things in the land of excess, we have fallen in love with the wrong kind of carbs. This was demonstrated by the selection of the worst restaurant dish in the United States a few years ago. David Zinczenko, the editor-in-chief of *Men's Health*, named Outback Steakhouse's Aussie Cheese Fries as the worst offender. Combined with a side of ranch dressing, this dish contains a staggering 240 grams of carbohydrates, more than a day's worth of calories at 2,900, and an artery-clogging 182 grams of fat.[1] All this in a dish that is supposed to be a preamble to the main course! Chili's Awesome Blossom onion outdoes these fries in the carb and fat categories, with 194 grams and 203 grams, respectively, plus a whopping 2,710 calories.[2]

It is easy to find bad carbs—they're everywhere! In the same way restaurants have taken unhealthy portions to new heights, manufacturers have undermined the purpose of healthy food. Manufacturers have taken the best of nature—fruits, vegetables, potatoes, sugarcane, corn, wheat, rice, and other grains—and processed and refined them by milling, pressing, squeezing, cooking, and separating whole foods into parts. Their procedures turn natural foods into man-made nightmares. Instead of fruit, we get processed, pasteurized juice, jams, pastries, and the like. Instead of sugarcane and corn, we end up with white sugar and sodas containing fattening, high-fructose corn syrup. Instead of whole-wheat bread, we get white bread, crackers, pasta, highly processed cereals, buns, bagels, pretzels, cakes, or muffins. And instead of brown rice or wild rice, we get white rice and rice cakes.

Bad Habits

Such processed habits are one reason that in recent years carbohydrates have received a bad rap. I have met countless individuals who during their initial appointments with me preached about the detriments of all carbs because that's what they had learned from past dieting experiences. They had climbed on board the high-protein diet train and weren't about to get off—even though such regimens had damaged their health. At times it was downright funny how adamantly they swore off carbs, as if touching them would instantly add a pound or two. The problem was, they couldn't sustain the no-carb approach for long. That is why they were in my office, weighing more than before starting their diet.

The National Institutes of Health recommends that 45 to 65 percent of our daily energy intake come from carbohydrates, with 25 to 35 percent of energy coming from fats and only 15 to 35 percent from proteins.[3] The American Diabetes Association also recommends 45 to 60 grams of carbohydrates in each meal, preferably from healthy whole grains. For diabetic and obese patients, I believe this is too many carbohydrates and too much grain. I believe excessive carbohydrates and grains are one of the main reasons for our obesity epidemic as well as our epidemic of type 2 diabetes. I typically recommend about 40 percent of daily calories come from low-glycemic carbohydrates, 30 percent from lean proteins, and 25 to 30 percent from healthy fats.

Have you ever wondered why there aren't more restaurants and fast-food chains touting natural carbs, such as whole-grain breads, steel-cut oats, whole fruits, broccoli, asparagus, beans, peas, or legumes? First, because these carbs are more filling—meaning customers rarely overeat them and are less likely to purchase other items on the menu. Second, these types of carbs do not have as long a shelf life—which should make you wonder what exactly is being put in the bad carbs to make them last so long.

The Tortoise and the Hare

Many people are familiar with the old story about the tortoise and the hare. The hare races ahead but fails to reach the finish line, while the slow but steady tortoise eventually passes him and wins the race. When it comes to how your body processes carbohydrates, the race that takes place within you is reminiscent of this classic fable. In this chapter I will take a look at two main types of carbohydrates: "tortoise carbs" and "hare carbs."

Before going further, I should explain that I am not talking about simple carbs vs. complex carbs, which are two common categories of carbs. Instead I will call low-glycemic carbs the "tortoise" and high-glycemic carbs the "hare."

Unfortunately, most of the carbohydrates overweight and obese people consume are not the kinds that assist with weight loss. Instead they are high-glycemic "hare carbs," which cause the blood sugar to rise rapidly. As I have already alluded to, this starts a chain of events that trap people in a fat-storage mode and prevent them from losing weight and reversing diabetes. The underlying cycle of hare carbs is obvious enough: the faster you absorb the carbs, the higher your insulin level rises, the more weight you gain, and the more diseases you develop, especially prediabetes and diabetes.

Welcome to the dark side of carbohydrates, where restaurant menus, grocery-store shelves, and home pantries overflow with highly pro-cessed, high-glycemic carbs. This romance with processed foods, such as breads, potatoes, and other grains, is one of the main reasons we see diabetes increasing at alarming rates. Yet it doesn't have to be this way. Better choices of high-fiber "tortoise-like" bread will pay dividends.

> ### RULE OF THUMB: BREADS
>
> The more processed and refined bread is, the less fiber it contains—and, ultimately, the less filling it is. Look for brands that contain at least 3 grams of fiber per slice. I also recommend double-fiber breads and sprouted breads.

The best choices of bread are the sprouted loaves found in most health food stores. I personally choose Ezekiel bread, which is made of the sprouts of wheat, barley, and other grains. It contains fewer calories than white bread, less than one-third the sodium, about half as many carbs, half the fat, and more than three times the fiber.

Remember, even if breads at the supermarket are called whole-grain breads, they also may contain sugar and hydrogenated fats and are pro-cessed in such a way that they still have fairly high glycemic indexes. Therefore if my diabetic patients request bread, I recommend that they have small amounts of sprouted bread in the morning or at lunch. I find that it tastes better when toasted. You can find Ezekiel bread in many grocery stores' frozen food section or online. The new double-fiber breads are a step in the right direction, but I still prefer the sprouted breads.

Carbohydrate and Sugar Addicts

When people crave highly processed carbohydrates, they are actually craving sugars. More often than not they are hooked on sugar. The diges-tive system quickly turns those highly processed carbs into sugar, which is rapidly absorbed into the bloodstream. This, in turn, spikes insulin, which drives the sugar into the cells and tissues. In only a few hours, when the cells in the hypothalamus sense inadequate sugar, appetite returns as the brain communicates that it needs a new "fix."

If you think I am going overboard with the drug addiction analogy, here's proof that I am not: Sugar and highly processed carbs release natural opioids in the brain. Your brain has opioid receptors. The phrase "runner's high" gets its name from the euphoric sensation that occurs when physical activity stimulates the brain to form endorphins. These neurotransmitters are similar in molecular structure to morphine, though much milder. They activate the brain's pleasure center.

Like exercise, sugars and highly processed carbohydrates are also able to trigger the release of such endorphins—which is why we call the result a "sugar high" or "sugar rush." Most people are unconsciously stimulating the pleasure centers in their brains by having a hit of sugar, white bread, muffin, bagel, doughnut, soda, or something similar. This is proof of how easy it is to become a sugar or carbohydrate addict; we are naturally programmed this way.

This opioid effect—and our natural inclination for it—has even been verified in infants. At Johns Hopkins University, researchers studied one- to three-day-old infants to observe their response to sugar. These babies were each placed in a bassinet for five minutes. When they began to whimper or cry, researchers gave them either a small amount of sugar in water or just plain water. They discovered that those who received sugar water stopped crying, while the plain water did nothing to stop the crying.[4]

In addition to activating opioid receptors, sugar and highly processed carbs also have a physiologically calming affect because of the release of serotonin in the brain. When the brain's serotonin level increases after you have eaten sweets or a refined starch, within twenty to thirty minutes you typically experience significant emotional relief. This also suppresses your appetite, improves your mood, helps you relax, makes you sleep better, and contributes to an overall feeling of well-being. Meanwhile, your body is programmed to store fat, all the while craving the next intake of feel-good but highly processed carbs.

Tortoise Carbs

Over the years I have attended a few financial seminars on investing. At almost every one the financial expert used the tortoise-and-hare analogy to show how long-term investing always wins out in the end. Though some investors manage to beat the odds by playing the market for short-term gains, it is undoubtedly the slow and steady, "in it for the long haul" investors who wind up with greater earnings. Because of this, these instructors hardly spent any time talking about next year's hottest stocks. Instead they offered plenty of advice on how to find those stocks or mutual funds that were consistent winners.

When it comes to weight-loss success, "tortoise carbs" are like long-term investments. These are the carbohydrates that slowly raise the blood sugar and enable you to lose weight and prevent or reverse diseases. We have spent the first part of this chapter discussing the lousy effects of "hare carbs." I will spend the rest of the chapter on natural, unprocessed carbs that can keep you healthy.

For starters, low-glycemic tortoise carbs can be broken down into the following groups:

- Vegetables
- Fruits
- Starches, such as whole-grain breads, whole-grain pasta, corn, oatmeal, unprocessed cereals, and sweet potatoes
- Dairy products, such as milk, yogurt, kefir, butter, and cheese
- Legumes, such as beans, peas, lentils, and peanuts
- Nuts and seeds

Even though most of these tortoise carbohydrates are healthy, it's still possible to choose the wrong types of starches and dairy or overeat low-glycemic starches, such as whole-grain bread and pasta. For this reason, and because there are other ways carbohydrates stall weight-loss efforts, it's important to incorporate the glycemic index and glycemic load principles we discussed in the last chapter.

Is It a Hare or a Tortoise?

The faster your body digests a carbohydrate, the faster it raises your blood sugar—and the higher the glycemic index value of that carb. This is what makes a carb a hare rather than a tortoise. Yet how exactly can you differentiate between the two? Here are a few traits that will help distinguish between a tortoise and a hare.

Fat content. With the exception of seeds, nuts, and dairy, most tortoise carbohydrates are low in fat. Fats are not an inherent evil as some diets claim. In fact, adequate amounts of fats in a meal are absolutely essential for keeping you satisfied longer and slowing the rate at which carbohydrates are broken down and released into the bloodstream—which is why most low-fat diets fail. This doesn't give you the license to down a bag of Doritos or other highly processed, high-fat carbohydrates just to get your fat content. Obviously you sabotage your weight-loss efforts when you do this.

Fiber content. Generally, a higher fiber content of a food slows down the absorption of sugar, making the carb a tortoise.

Form of starch. Certain starches, such as potatoes, white bread, and white rice contain amylopectin, which is a complex carbohydrate that the body rapidly absorbs and that usually raises one's blood sugar. However, some whole grains, beans, peas, legumes, and sweet potatoes contain another complex carb called amylose, which is digested more slowly and raises the blood sugar in a slower fashion as well. However, caution is needed with whole-wheat products since 75 percent is amylopectin and only 25 percent is amylose, which is absorbed more slowly. Many corn products, such as cornmeal, corn pasta, and corn flakes, are digested fairly rapidly and therefore are considered hare carbohydrates (with a high glycemic index value). However, corn on the cob or frozen corn is digested more slowly and only gradually raises the blood sugar.

Ripeness. The riper the fruit, the faster it is absorbed. An example of this is the difference between yellow bananas and brown, spotted bananas. The latter raise the blood sugar much faster than regular yellow bananas since they are riper and have a higher sugar content.

Cooking. Most pasta can be either a tortoise carbohydrate or a hare carbohydrate, depending on how you cook it. If you cook it al dente, which means for about five or six minutes and still leaving it firm, it is typically a tortoise carbohydrate and has a low glycemic index value. If you cook it for a longer period of time to soften it, pasta becomes a hare carbohydrate with a high glycemic index value. Also, thicker pasta generally has a lower glycemic index value than thinner types of pasta, while whole-grain pasta is lower glycemic than refined white pasta. Again, I advise caution with all wheat products, even whole grain, since they have a higher glycemic load than many other carbohydrates.

Milling type. A finely ground grain is a hare carbohydrate and has a higher glycemic index value than coarsely ground grain, which has a higher fiber content and thus is a tortoise.

Protein content. The higher the protein content of a food, the more it helps prevent a rapid rise in blood sugar and makes the food more likely to be lower glycemic. Thus it is a tortoise carbohydrate.

The Less Sugar, the Better

We have already talked about the different types of carbohydrates; now let's briefly discuss sugar. Unfortunately, statistics show that Americans have become too familiar with this elemental substance. The average American consumes about 156 pounds of sugar a year![5] Let's put that into perspective: A single 12-ounce can of carbonated soda typically contains 8 to 10 teaspoons of sugar.[6] If you drink soft drinks throughout the day, you can see how this added sugar intake quickly adds up. And it's even worse for teenagers, who consume a daily average of 28 teaspoons a day, compared to 21 teaspoons for adults.[7]

Most everyone knows the foods that are high in sugar—desserts, sodas, candy, cookies, cakes, pies, doughnuts, and the like. The general public is a little less knowledgeable about those starchy foods that, while not touted as high-sugar items, usually have high glycemic values. I cannot stress enough how important avoiding sugar is to losing weight and reversing diabetes-related problems. I realize this isn't easy. As I mentioned earlier, sugar often triggers the release of endorphins, which gives us a sugar high—and acts like a drug, leading to cravings for more and more sugar.

NATIONAL SUGAR HIGH

In the early 1980s roughly one in seven Americans was obese and almost six million were diabetic. By the early 2000s, when national sugar consumption hit its peak, one in three Americans were obese and fourteen million were diabetic.[8]

The trouble is that eating sugar programs our body for weight gain. It also makes us more susceptible to insulin resistance, metabolic syndrome, type 2 diabetes, and heart disease. Excess sugar also triggers free-radical reactions in our bodies, leading to chronic disease, accelerated aging, and plaque formation in our arteries. Especially in diabetics, excess sugar can cause glycation, where sugar molecules react with protein molecules to cause wrinkled skin and damaged tissues. The bottom line is that—contrary to those images projected in TV advertisements—too much sugar does not produce a pretty face or body. Eat too much, and you will end up flabby and wrinkled.

Use Safe Sweeteners

For several years the dieting gimmick was (and to a degree still is) simply replacing these excess sugars with artificial sweeteners. There are plenty of sweeteners available, the most widely known being aspartame and sucralose. I do not recommend either one of these. (For detailed reasons on why neither of these work, see *The Seven Pillars of Health*.) There are, however, three natural sweeteners that are safe and low glycemic.

UNNATURALLY SWEET

Splenda, which is made by turning sugar into a chlorocarbon, is approximately 600 times sweeter than sugar.[9]

Stevia

This is an herbal sweetener with no calories and a glycemic index value of zero. It is my favorite; I use the liquid form in my coffee and tea. In this form it is very sweet—approximately 200 times sweeter than sugar. Because of this, you only need to use a tiny amount. Stevia is also available in granulated form. Products such as Truvia contain granulated stevia in convenient single-serving packets and can be found in most grocery stores. If powdered or liquid stevia tastes too sweet, I suggest trying the granulated form, which is more like the consistency and sweetness of sugar.

AGAVE NECTAR AND HIGH-FRUCTOSE CORN SYRUP

In spite of what you may have heard, agave nectar is not made from the sap of the agave plant but from the starch of the agave root bulb. The agave root contains starch—similar to that in corn or rice—and a complex carbohydrate called inulin, which is made up of fructose.

Similar to the way cornstarch is converted into high-fructose corn syrup (HFCS), agave starch goes through a chemical process that converts the starch into a fructose-rich syrup—anywhere from 70 percent fructose and higher, according to several agave nectar websites.

That means that the refined fructose in agave nectar is even more concentrated than the fructose in HFCS. For comparison, the HFCS used in sodas is 55 percent refined fructose.[10] For this reason I do not recommend using agave as an alternative to sugar, syrup, or other sweeteners.

Xylitol

A sugar alcohol, xylitol also has a very low glycemic index value. It also kills bacteria and prevents dental cavities. I have used xylitol as a nose drop to treat patients with sinus infections. It tastes just like sugar, with no aftertaste, and is a good substitute for sugar for cooking or baking. However, because it is a sugar alcohol, some individuals may experience bloating, gas, diarrhea, or other gastrointestinal issues when using xylitol in larger quantities. Because it is a natural sweetener and our bodies do produce it, I still recommend using it, but initially in very low doses to avoid any GI disturbance.

Chicory

Chicory is a natural sweetener that usually contains chicory root, which is a probiotic food that helps improve your GI function. In addition to supporting your weight-loss efforts, chicory does not promote tooth decay. It is available at retail stores like Whole Foods and many health food stores. I find it a wonderful, natural alternative to sugar and harmful artificial sweeteners without the intense sweet aftertaste that deters some people from using stevia.

Chapter 11

WHAT YOU NEED TO KNOW ABOUT FIBER AND FATS

Earlier I mentioned growing up in the South on a diet that featured fried everything—with gravy. Yet I can still hear that short one-sentence lecture from my mother that, ironically, stood at the opposite end of the nutrition spectrum: "You need your roughage!"

Roughage is a catch-all term for fiber-rich food, drawing its name from the propensity of such foods to easily work their way through your system. Though often a source of bathroom humor, fiber plays a crucial role in the battle against diabetes. Ironically, while Americans are shorting their diets when it comes to fiber, they also ingest way too much fat—so much that many healthy-eating proponents have gone to the other extreme and condemned all kinds and types of fat. Don't listen to them. Fat is as essential to a balanced diet as getting adequate amounts of fiber.

Fantastic Fiber

Another important way you can seek to battle and reverse diabetes through nutrition is to increase the amount of fiber in your diet. Soluble fiber is a key weapon in helping control diabetes. It slows down the digestion and absorption of carbohydrates. It also slows glucose uptake and thus lowers the glycemic index of your meal. This in turn lowers the amount of insulin that is secreted by the pancreas, which is very beneficial for those with type 2 diabetes. Soluble fiber has also been shown over the years through numerous studies to effectively lower blood sugar levels.

How does it do all of these things? Soluble fiber actually swells many times its original size as it binds to the water in your stomach and small intestine to form a viscous gel that not only slows down the absorption of glucose but also induces a sense of satiety (fullness) and reduces your body's absorption of calories.

Studies conducted by James W. Anderson, MD, of the University of

Kentucky showed that high-fiber diets lowered insulin requirements an average of 38 percent in people with type 1 diabetes and 97 percent in people with type 2 diabetes. This means that almost all of the people suffering from type 2 diabetes who followed Dr. Anderson's high-fiber diet were able to lower or stop taking insulin and other diabetes medications and still maintain a healthy blood sugar level. Additionally, these results lasted up to fifteen years.[1]

INCREASING FIBER IN YOUR DIET

Try the following five ideas to increase the fiber in your diet:

1. Eat at least five servings of fruit and vegetables each day. Fruit and vegetables that are high in fiber include:

- Brussels sprouts
- Peas
- Beans (all types)
- Broccoli
- Parsnips
- Spinach
- Legumes
- Berries
- Raw carrots
- Lentils

2. Replace breads and cereals made from refined flours with sprouted breads and high-fiber cereals. Eat brown rice instead of white rice. Some examples of these good foods:

- Walnuts, almonds, and macadamia nuts
- Old-fashioned steel-cut oatmeal or high-fiber instant oatmeal
- Brown rice
- Flaxseeds, chia seeds, hemp seeds, pumpkin seeds, and sunflower seeds
- Ezekiel Bread or other type of sprouted bread

3. Eat high-fiber cereal for breakfast. Check labels on the packages for the amounts of dietary fiber. Some cereals may have less fiber than you think. Some good choices are Fiber One and All Bran with Extra Fiber.

4. Eat cooked beans, peas, or lentils a few times a week.

5. Take capsules of PGX fiber (two to three capsules with 16 ounces of water before each meal).

If you have diabetes, a significant amount of the carbohydrate calories you eat should come from vegetables, including peas, beans, lentils, and legumes. Those vegetables typically contain large amounts of soluble fiber. The more soluble fiber in your diet, the better your blood sugar control. Water-soluble fibers are found in oat bran, seeds such as psyllium (the primary ingredient in Metamucil), fruit (especially Granny Smith apples and berries), vegetables, beans, and nuts.

Many foods contain dietary fiber. Eating foods that are high in fiber can relieve some diabetes problems, help lower your cholesterol, and even prevent heart disease and certain types of cancer.

Fiber is also one of the most important carbohydrates for weight control. It lowers a food's glycemic index and usually prevents the sugar spike and elevated insulin levels that occur with high-glycemic foods. Even high-glycemic foods, such as sugars, cakes, pies, and cookies, can be turned into medium-glycemic foods by eating sufficient fiber. As I tell my patients, "Fiber covers a multitude of dietary sins!"

Fiber also keeps you full and satisfied for longer periods of time. It significantly reduces your appetite by filling your stomach and slowing down the rate at which your body absorbs sugars into the bloodstream. Eating high-fiber foods also takes longer to chew and dramatically slows down the act of eating, which helps prevent you from consuming excessive calories before the satiety center in your brain realizes it. (One note: you should eat fiber with meals in order to prevent rapid rises in blood sugar.)

Unfortunately, most Americans do not eat enough fiber. Though the numbers vary with age, the Institute of Medicine recommends that men consume about 38 grams of fiber a day and women around 25 grams. However, according to the institute, the average man and woman in the United States currently consumes less than half that amount.[2]

To get its full benefits, it helps to know the difference between two major types of fiber: soluble and insoluble. Most dietary fiber is indigestible and is excreted in the stool. Although both types of fiber slow down the rate at which carbohydrates are digested and enter the bloodstream, there are some noticeable differences.

IT'S ALL ABOUT FIBER

Since only 5 percent of Americans consume an adequate amount of daily fiber, women hoping to lose weight should concentrate more on getting enough fiber rather than following through with low-carb, low-fat, or high-protein diets. This was confirmed by a study of more than 4,500 people, which also discovered that women on a low-fiber, high-fat diet have an increased risk of being overweight or obese.[3]

Soluble fiber. This type dissolves in the intestines. Foods high in soluble fiber include legumes, beans, peas, lentils, apples, citrus food, oats, barley, flaxseeds, and psyllium seeds and husks. Soluble fiber forms a sticky, gummy substance as it passes through the intestines. Acting like a sponge, it soaks up and traps excessive cholesterol, sugar, and toxins and excretes them. Soluble fiber helps you lose weight, decreases your appetite, and lowers cholesterol and blood sugar. The latter reduces your risk of heart disease.

Insoluble fiber. Derived from the cell walls of plants, this type consists mainly of cellulose, which is indigestible and does not dissolve in the intestines. It is found mainly in whole grains, wheat bran, and in lower amounts in fruits and vegetables. Insoluble fiber adds bulk to the stool, relieves constipation, and helps clean the colon. It aids in controlling the appetite and prevents constipation and diverticulitis.

Both soluble and insoluble fiber help control your appetite, lower cholesterol levels, stabilize blood sugar, decrease your risk of chronic disease, improve bowel function, and assist with weight loss.

One word of caution: When adding fiber to your diet, make small changes over a period of time to help prevent bloating, cramping, or gas. Start by adding one of the items listed above to your diet, then wait several days or a week before making another change. If one change doesn't seem to work for you, try a different one. It's important to drink more fluids when you increase the amount of fiber you eat. Drink at least two additional glasses of water a day when you increase your fiber intake.

The Fat Truth

For decades physicians, nutritionists, dietitians, and other health authorities have blamed fats for every diet-related problem under the sun: the obesity epidemic, elevated cholesterol, and heart disease. It's as if someone devised a master plan to take a single "truth" and transform an entire nation's dietary mind-set. The premise: all fats make you fat.

As a result, people flocked like lemmings to anything labeled "low-fat" or "no fat." Everyone started going on low-fat diets, cooking from low-fat cookbooks, and eating low-fat crackers, low-fat chips, low-fat ice cream, and low-fat cookies. Americans decreased their consumption of fat from 45 percent of daily caloric intake in the mid-1960s to 38 percent in the 1980s to approximately 35 percent of calories in the mid-1990s.[4] One problem, though: we kept on gaining weight.

In fact, obesity has skyrocketed in this country to unparalleled proportions while the average weight of Americans has steadily increased too. If fats are supposed to make you fat, then why has cutting back on them made Americans fatter? Something doesn't add up. The truth: fats don't necessarily make you fat. There are bad fats that put on weight, but there are also good fats that enable you to lose weight. The good fats help prevent heart disease, lower triglycerides, and ward off a multitude of diseases. The bottom line is that too much of any fat—good or bad—will make you fat.

Still, fats are vital for good health. Among their many roles, they provide fuel for your cells. A fatty cell membrane, composed primarily of polyunsaturated and saturated fats, surrounds each of the trillions of cells in your body. Saturated fats provide a rigid support for the cell membrane. Polyunsaturated fats add flexibility to the cell membranes and allow the transfer of nutrients inside cells and waste products to pass to the outside. These cell membranes need a proper balance of both.

Likewise, we need a balance of fats in our diet to help with the absorption of fat-soluble vitamins, including vitamins A, D, E, and K. And we need fats to produce hormones that regulate inflammation, blood clotting, and muscle contraction. Approximately 60 percent of your brain is composed of fat. You need cholesterol to make brain cells, and most cholesterol comes from saturated fats. Fats make up the coverings that surround and protect nerves. They help to satisfy hunger for extended periods.

Types of Fats

Fats can be broken down into two main types: saturated and unsaturated. Within the unsaturated fats category are three smaller groupings, which are omega-6 fats, omega-9 fats, and omega-3 fats.

Omega-3 and omega-6 fats are polyunsaturated fats, while omega-9 fats are monounsaturated fats. Only two fats within these subcategories are required for health: linoleic acid, an omega-6 fatty acid, and alpha-linolenic acid, an omega-3 fatty acid. Our bodies are capable of producing all other types of fats by consuming these two. That leaves omega-9 fats left out in the rain, since they are considered nonessential.

Since all this may leave you scratching your head, I have categorized fats into three main categories: bad fats, good fats, and fats that can be good or bad, depending on the amount ingested.

Bad Fats

Trans fats

These are man-made fats, such as those present in margarine, shortening, most commercially baked foods, many deep-fried foods, many commercial peanut butters, and processed foods such as crackers, cookies, cakes, pies, and breads. The problem with trans fats is that they are synthetic and toxic.

They are inflammatory fats that raise cholesterol, form plaque in the arteries, and increase the risk of obesity, heart disease, type 2 diabetes, and cancer.

How bad are trans fats? Open up a tub of margarine and set it outside. Typically, even insects won't go near it. So how in the world did we wind up putting this substance in the majority of our foods? Good question. After being developed in Germany and mass-produced in England, trans fats came to America in 1911 with the introduction of Crisco. To boost sales, the company gave away cookbooks in which every recipe required this hydrogenated shortening.[5] By the advent of World War II—with butter in short supply—trans fats became ingrained in our culture. Processed food companies had the perfect fat. It was cheap, wouldn't spoil, and had an extremely long shelf life.

My, how the times have changed. In January 2007, the US Food and Drug Administration (FDA) almost banned Crisco. Rather than fold up shop, though, the product's maker agreed to reformulate its shortening to contain zero trans fats per serving.[6] This fell more in line with the government's general recommendation to either not eat trans fats or only in very small quantities. The reasons go beyond adding pounds. By consuming trans fats, your cells and cell membranes become hydrogenated or partially hydrogenated, growing rigid and stiff.

FOODS THAT OFTEN HAVE TRANS FATS

- Fast foods
- Packaged foods
- Frozen foods
- Candy and cookies
- Baked goods
- Chips and crackers
- Toppings, dips, and condiments
- Soups
- Margarine and butter
- Breakfast foods

Researchers found out that women who consumed the most trans fats—about 3 percent of daily energy, or about 7 grams of fat—over a fourteen-year period were twice as likely to develop heart disease than those who ate the least amounts.[7] Overall, experts agree that each gram of trans fat consumed increases the risk of heart disease by approximately 20 percent. In addition, trans fats further obesity risks by increasing insulin resistance and the size of fat cells, which in turn enables them to store more fat.

The public is slowly catching on to the dangers. Beginning in 2006, the FDA mandated labeling of all foods containing trans fats. Fortunately, many fast-food restaurants and processed food companies dropped their use. But that does not mean we can celebrate. When Dunkin' Donuts shed trans fats in 2007, they switched to a blend of palm, soybean, and cottonseed oils[8] (still not a health food). Check fast-food offerings and others on store shelves. Learn to read labels, and avoid foods containing hydrogenated or partially hydrogenated oils or trans fats.

Refined polyunsaturated fats

This is another type of bad fat that causes weight gain. The majority of Americans consume excessive amounts. They are found in most salad dressings and commercial vegetable oils, such as sunflower, safflower, corn, cottonseed, or soybean oil. These omega-6 fats have been refined and heated to high temperatures. Thus they are typically high in dangerous lipid peroxides, which trigger inflammation. These fats are also associated with weight gain because of their tendency to increase insulin resistance.

READ YOUR FOOD LABELS

Since foods can still contain up to 0.5 grams of trans fats per serving while being labeled as having zero trans fats, the best way to avoid consuming trans fats unawares is to look for the words "partially hydrogenated" or "shortening" on the label or ingredient list. If you find either, don't eat the product!

Deep-fried foods

Deep-fried foods, such as french fries, onion rings, fried chicken, deep-fried fish, fried corn or potato chips, and hush puppies, are loaded with inflammatory fats. Imagine taking a sponge, dropping it in water, and wringing all of the water out. That is similar to what you are doing when you toss french fries, onion rings, or chicken into a deep fryer. That food is literally soaking up the grease and fat. Instead of wringing it out of a sponge, you put it in your mouth. In the process your body is being programmed to store fat. Parents who regularly feed their children french fries, deep-fried chicken, and fried chicken strips are unknowingly setting up their children for a life-long struggle with obesity.

MISLEADING LABELS

On January 1, 2006, all packaged foods sold in the United States began to list trans fat content on their nutrition labels. But under FDA regulations, "if the serving contains less than 0.5 gram [of trans fat], the content, when declared, shall be expressed as zero."[9] That means you could eat several cookies, each with 0.4 grams of trans fat, and end up eating several grams of trans fats even though the label says zero!

Fats That May Be Good or Bad

Some fats can be good or bad, depending on the amount ingested. These include saturated fats and unrefined omega-6 fats, which are polyunsaturated fats.

Saturated fats

Are these good or bad? It depends on the type and amount consumed. Saturated fats are found primarily in animal products, including meat such as beef, pork, lamb, and poultry. More precisely, they lie in animal fat—the visible fat around a piece of steak or marbled fat mixed with meat, which makes prime rib and rib eye steaks so juicy. Finally, saturated fats are found in poultry skins; dairy products such as butter, cream, and cheese; and a few vegetable oils—palm oil, palm kernel oil, and coconut oil.

Thousands of studies prove that excessive intake of saturated fats is associated with an increase in LDL cholesterol (the bad kind) and increased risk of atherosclerosis and cardiovascular disease.

Many people are unaware of the many types of saturated fats. The short-chain variety is present in coconut oil and palm kernel oil, both of which are excellent sources of fuel for the body and easily digestible. These fatty acids are healthier and less likely to elevate cholesterol levels (unless consumed in excess). Coconut oil also contains lauric acid, which helps immune system function and is present in breast milk.

The next type includes medium-chain triglycerides (MCTs). These are also found in coconut oil and palm kernel oil. These fats are digested and utilized differently than other saturated fats. They first go to the liver and are rapidly converted to energy. Athletes use these fats quite frequently; they produce immediate energy, and the body typically does not store them as fat. MCTs also help increase the metabolic rate. Yet be aware MCTs can be stored as fat, especially with too many calories and a lack of exercise.

The worse types of saturated fats are the long-chain saturated fats, especially in such fatty cuts as most hamburger meat, ribs, rib eye, prime rib, sausage, and bacon. All are associated with raising LDL cholesterol. Long-chain saturated fats are present in all meat and high-fat dairy products such as butter and cheese.

Saturated fats should make up approximately 5 to 10 percent of your food intake. However, if you have elevated levels of cholesterol, the National Cholesterol Education Program recommends no more than 7 percent of your daily calories come from saturated fat.[10] When you consistently consume more than 10 percent of total calories as saturated fat, you increase your risk of high cholesterol, atherosclerosis, insulin resistance, and weight gain.

Cutting back

So how do you lower your intake? Choose extra-lean cuts of meat and low-fat or nonfat dairy products, remove poultry skins, trim off all visible fats, and limit red meat to two or three times a week (a maximum of 18 ounces a week). I recommend more turkey and chicken breast, which are typically low in saturated fats—provided they are free range and organic. I also like fish, low in mercury, but be careful to avoid farm-raised varieties. Fish with low mercury levels according to the FDA include anchovies, butterfish, cod, flatfish, haddock, hake, herring, jacksmelt, mackerel, perch (ocean), pollack, salmon (canned), salmon (fresh/frozen), sardine, tilapia, trout, tuna (especially tongol tuna), whitefish, and whiting. Women should limit portion sizes of these proteins to 2 to 6 ounces per meal while men should aim for between 3 and 8 ounces.

This may seem like a small amount, especially to men accustomed to huge steaks. No matter how much you love steak, though, it is loaded with saturated fats that lock you into obesity, often via insulin resistance. Remember that free-range, grass-fed, or organically fed animals—buffalo, bison, or elk—typically have much less saturated fat than grain-fed animals.

Omega-6 fats

We all need small amounts of unrefined omega-6 fats on a daily basis for good health. For example, everyone requires linoleic acid, but most people take in excessive amounts, often in the form of salad dressings and refined oils (corn, soy, sunflower, safflower oil, cottonseed oil). Many processed foods, fast foods, and restaurant foods are extremely high in refined omega-6 fatty acids. The recommended ratio of omega-6 fatty acids to omega-3 fatty acids should be approximately four to one. Currently, most Americans consume about a twenty-to-one ratio![11] Omega-3 fats suppress inflammation; omega-6 fats promote it.

Instead of refined omega-6 fats, choose small amounts of expeller- or cold-pressed oils: extra-virgin olive oil, high oleic safflower, and sunflower oil, which are high in monounsaturated fats. Healthy sources of omega-6 fats include most seeds and nuts. Although seeds and nuts are high in fat, they are also high in fiber, which is filling, satisfying, and prevents some fat absorption. Keep in mind that an excessive consumption of even good omega-6 fats can cause weight gain, and they promote inflammation, which is at the root of most chronic diseases, including obesity and type 2 diabetes. As always, the key is moderation.

Healthy Fats

GLA

Gamma linolenic acid (GLA) is produced in the body from linoleic acid (LA). Think of GLA as a "super LA." It is a beneficial fatty acid that helps to decrease inflammation. Oils that contain GLA include borage, evening primrose, and black currant seed oil. Unfortunately, GLA is not found in most foods. Even though LA is an essential fatty acid, many individuals are unable to convert LA to GLA and are thus at a higher risk of developing inflammation, impaired immune response, allergies, and insulin resistance. This also means that the risk of weight gain and fat storage increases due to their bodies' inability to produce adequate amounts of GLA.

Most people who naturally produce GLA are young and healthy. This is because the body's ability to convert LA to GLA is impaired by excessive amounts of stress; the intake of trans fats, saturated fats, and omega-6 fats; and aging.

Omega-3 fats

Without getting into too many details, it is important to explain a bit more about omega-3 fats, since they are often automatically associated with fish. There are three types: alpha-linolenic acid (ALA), found in flaxseeds and flaxseed oil; eicosapentaenoic acid (EPA), found in cold-water fish; and docosahexaenoic acid (DHA), found in cold-water fish and some algae. Approximately 99 percent of Americans are deficient in these healthy fats.

Unfortunately, many individuals are unable to produce EPA and DHA from ALA because of impairments in the enzyme making this conversion, usually from stress, aging, and excessive intake of trans, saturated, and omega-6 fats. Therefore, even if you are eating a lot of flaxseed oil and flax-seeds, you still may not have adequate amounts of EPA and DHA.

Omega-3 fats, particularly EPA and DHA, have many benefits. They decrease inflammation, lower triglycerides, assist in preventing and treating heart disease, support the immune system, and prompt the release of stored fat. The best sources of omega-3 are fatty fish, such as salmon, mackerel, herring, and sardines. Quality fish oil supplements are good alternatives.

A diet with sufficient amounts of omega-3s will usually prevent and may eventually reverse insulin resistance. These fats help the body shed abdominal weight. Good fats in the form of fatty fish or fish oil capsules are a must for anyone wanting to lose weight in this region. And omega-3 fats also decrease the risk of developing diabetes.

I mentioned earlier the benefits of choosing free-range, grass-fed, or organically fed animals. Animals that are typically grain fed include cows, pigs, and even chickens. Their meat usually contains a very low concentration of omega-3 fatty acids and significantly higher amounts of omega-6 fatty acids. Grain-fed meat is also typically high in saturated fats. However, free-range or grass-fed animals typically have much higher concentrations of omega-3 fats in their tissues and lower levels of omega-6 and saturated fats.

Monounsaturated fats

These are also good fats. Certain Mediterranean diets consume up to 40 percent of their daily calories from monounsaturated fats, primarily in the form of olive oil. In what became known as the Seven Countries Study, Ancel Keys, PhD, and other researchers studied more than twelve thousand men between the ages of forty and fifty from 1958 to 1964.

Keys discovered that those in the Mediterranean groups had the lowest mortality rates from all causes. Greek men had the lowest mortality rate overall and the lowest rate of heart disease. Finnish men had the highest rate of heart disease. They consumed almost 40 percent of calories from fats, with more than 50 percent coming from saturated fats. Among other things, the study proved that olive oil and other monounsaturated fats are extremely healthy fats.[12]

Monounsaturated fats are in the omega-9 category and are considered non-essential, since the body can make them from other fats. Regardless, monounsaturated fats are extremely healthy and are anti-inflammatory, helping lower LDL cholesterol without decreasing good HDL cholesterol. They also help to support the immune system and aid weight loss.

Foods high in monounsaturated fats include olives, olive oil, avocados, almonds, hazelnuts, pecans, cashews, macadamia nuts, peanuts, peanut oil, Brazilian nuts, sesame seeds, sunflower seeds, pumpkin seeds, and canola oil.

Since most fats are inflammatory and promote insulin resistance, the root cause of diabetes, I have my diabetic patients choose mainly omega-3 fats and monounsaturated fats, which are both anti-inflammatory.

FATS THAT MAKE YOU SKINNY

A study from Brigham and Women's Hospital in Boston reveals why, for weight loss, a Mediterranean-style diet using olive oil trumps a traditional low-fat diet. Those on the latter limited fat intake to 20 percent of calories, while those on the Mediterranean diet could obtain 35 percent from olive oil, nuts, and other monounsaturated fats. After six months, both groups lost weight. Yet, after eighteen months, only 20 percent of those on the low-fat diet stuck with it and most regained weight. The majority of those on the Mediterranean diet not only stayed on it, but they also kept their pounds off.[13]

The Big Fat Problem

As mentioned at the beginning of this chapter, the majority of Americans consume approximately one-third of their total calories from fats. Even though this is a fairly safe amount, Americans continue to gain weight and suffer from an epidemic of being overweight and obese and of suffering from prediabetes and type 2 diabetes. For this reason I recommend approximately 25 to 30 percent of your total calorie intake as fats (making sure to choose good fats) in order to improve insulin resistance, decrease inflammation, and lose weight. I cannot stress enough the importance of both the type of fats and the ratio of fats consumed.

I suggest about 10 to 20 percent of your fat intake be monounsaturated fats and 5 to 10 percent polyunsaturated fats, with a four-to-one ratio of omega-6 to omega-3 fats. In other words, if 2.5 grams of your fats are omega-3 fats, consume 7.5 grams of omega-6 fats, with GLA being the best form of omega-6 fats. Finally, no more than 5 to 10 percent of fat intake should be saturated fats. I recommend avoiding all trans fats, fried foods, and refined omega-6 fats, such as most regular salad dressings.

Whenever I explain fats to patients, I say they simply need an oil change. You would not think of driving year after year without changing your car's oil because eventually you would ruin the engine. Our bodies are no different. We need the proper balance of healthy oils in our body for healthy cells, tissues, and organs. Fats are not evil; however, inflammatory fats such as trans fats, fried foods, omega-6 fats, and saturated fats make one more prone to develop insulin resistance and eventually prediabetes and diabetes. You can use the right proportion and amount of good fats to help you lose weight. Now go get an oil change—and don't forget the fiber.

Chapter 12

BEVERAGES: ARE YOU DRINKING YOUR WAY TO DIABETES?

Commercials have become such an integral part of American life that the year's most highly watched TV event—the Super Bowl—includes millions who tune in solely to review, critique, and rate the advertisements. The beverage makers who help drive this multimillion-dollar bonanza are also among the cleverest marketers. After stumbling in 2010, when only one of the top ten viewer-rated commercials featured a beverage (Budweiser), four of the top ten for the 2011 Super Bowl were produced by beer (Budweiser) and soft drink (Pepsi and Coca-Cola) companies.

I have to hand it to them. Whether it is optimistic youth harmonizing about a perfect world, sports announcers analyzing the "Bud Bowl," a partying bull terrier named Spuds MacKenzie, or polar bears watching the aurora borealis while sipping Coke, for decades the beverage industry has created ingenious ways of shaping public perceptions. From hilarious beer commercials to ridiculous yet always memorable soft-drink ads, marketers have persuaded Americans they can purchase fun, popularity, or physical prowess in a can.

However, they are better at distracting people with fond memories and good feelings about their product than informing you of their content and potential health hazards. Here are a few truths about these sugar-charged, calorie-laden drinks that are a gateway to diabetes:

- A 12-ounce can of Coke Classic contains 140 calories and 39 grams (approximately 10 teaspoons) of sugar.
- A "healthy" bottle of Dole's Ruby Red Grapefruit juice packs in 63 grams of carbs (55 of them sugar, which is approximately 14 teaspoons of sugar) and 260 calories in a 15-ounce serving.
- A "diet" carbonated drink can possibly lead to greater weight gain than a regular soda.

Despite their drawbacks, we continue to guzzle their drinks, taking a toll on our nation's waistlines. According to the Beverage Marketing Corporation, the average person (adult or child) ingests approximately 192 gallons of liquid a year. That amounts to approximately 3.7 gallons a week, or half a gallon a day.[1] However, the problem doesn't lie so much in how much we are drinking but what we are drinking.

WHAT THE AVERAGE AMERICAN DRINKS[2]	
Type of Beverage	Percent of Total Consumption
Carbonated soft drinks	28.3
Beer	11.7*
Milk	10.9
Bottled water	10.7
Coffee	9.0
Fruit beverages	4.7
Tea	3.8

Total alcohol consumption was 13 percent, with wine at 1.2 percent and distilled spirits at 0.7 percent.

I emphasize drinking at least one quart of water each day. Yet look at the percentages of the types of beverages people consume. According to the above chart, 40 percent of all beverages consumed are carbonated soft drinks or alcoholic beverages. More than two-thirds are high calorie. We are literally drinking ourselves into obesity and drawing ourselves down the road toward diabetes, obesity, and other health problems.

Feeling Thirsty?

Why do we continue to guzzle extra calories and sugars with little thought of the consequences? Beyond the fruity flavors and "great taste, less filling" arguments, it starts with a basic force: thirst. Your thirst center is located in the brain. Thirst is the primary way your body signals you that you need to ingest more fluids. This is triggered by a decrease in blood volume or an increase of sodium in the blood. Drinking a beverage increases the blood volume and dilutes the sodium, thus quenching thirst.

However, for those trying to control their weight and reverse diabetes, many of these drinks do not curb the appetite or satisfy hunger. That is of little concern to beverage makers, who appeal to your need for satisfying your thirst with their drink. This is why near any grocery or convenience store you will typically find a massive billboard or poster showing a cool, refreshing drink. And why a refrigerated container stocked with ice-cold drinks stands near every checkout line.

When you absorb sugar or high-fructose corn syrup from a soda into your bloodstream—usually a rapid process—it spikes

> ### BIG GULPS
>
> The National Soft Drink Association reports that the average person consumes more than 600 12-ounce servings of soft drinks a year. While I stress drinking one to two quarts of water a day, males twelve to twenty-nine gulp down an astonishing 160-plus gallons a year. That amounts to almost two quarts of soft drinks daily.[3]

your blood sugar, causing a surge of insulin to be released from the pancreas. In turn, that eventually triggers the appetite. Soft drinks simultaneously quench thirst *and* trigger appetite, yet they cannot curb hunger. So what usually happens next? Within an hour or two, the average American is reaching for a high-calorie snack to raise his or her blood sugar. It's a vicious cycle, but one that endures.

The Soda Snare

This habit ensnares millions of people, like Anne. A forty-two-year-old accountant, when she came to see me she was prediabetic, and no wonder. She described starting her typical day with coffee and a bagel loaded with cream cheese. Around midmorning she drank a soda; for lunch she usually had a healthy soup with soda. At midafternoon she reached for another "pick me up" soda. At night she drank iced tea with a healthy meal. Although she worked out five days a week, always passed on desserts, and did not consume excessive calories, Anne couldn't lose weight. She felt even more frustrated looking at many slender coworkers, who even ate dessert but never seemed to put on weight.

After a while, she noticed that in place of sodas, they were drinking water and unsweetened tea. Anne could not bring herself to go cold turkey, so she compromised and switched to diet soda. Within a few months she had gained 5 pounds. Talk about frustrating! By the time she scheduled an appointment, Anne was 35 pounds overweight and about to give up. Upon taking her dietary and beverage history, it did not take long to figure out the source of her problems.

When I switched Anne to water with lemon and unsweetened green tea and adjusted her food intake, she began to lose weight. Within six months she had lost 35 pounds and her blood sugar was normal.

Diet Sodas

Anne's case is more common than you might think. I have counseled hundreds of exasperated patients who thought their weight loss solution lay in switching from regular soda to diet. "After all, there are barely any calories in them, right?" they would ask. Somewhere between the first reduced-calorie drink and the emergence of artificial sweeteners, we believed we could lose weight by changing to diet soda.

A handful of studies show the opposite. These reports indicate that drinking diet sodas can cause weight gain. One study covering eight years' worth of data found that drinking one or two cans of soda each day led to a 32.8 percent greater chance of becoming overweight. When diet sodas were consumed in place of regular ones at the same rate, the risk increased to a whopping 54.5 percent.[4]

I'll be honest: the reasons are not yet fully known. Researchers have yet to understand the direct connection between diet drinks and weight gain. What we do know is that somehow diet sodas trigger the body to store fat.

DIET DRINKS AND METABOLIC SYNDROME

A recent study of more than 9,500 people found that those who consumed at least one can of diet soda per day had a 34 percent higher chance of developing metabolic syndrome than those who did not drink diet sodas.[5]

Some researchers believe that the tremendous sweetness of these artificial substances, typically two hundred to two thousand times sweeter than sugar, causes users to crave more sweets.

In addition, diet sodas are most likely increasing insulin levels and setting up people for increased hunger and fat storage. This is exactly what Anne experienced.

As the Soda Grows (So Grows the Waistline)

There is another factor to the connection between growing waistlines and soda, whether regular or diet. In the 1950s Coke came in 6-ounce bottles. Now "small" cans are twice that size, and the standard bottle is 20 ounces, which represents 2.5 servings. That means when you examine the per-serving information, you have to multiply by 2.5 to gauge the bottle's full impact.

The Center for Science in the Public Interest places the average daily soda consumption for adults at about 18 ounces of soda, with per-capita consumption nearly tripling between 1977 and 2000.[6] It obviously does not help that most fast-food restaurants and convenience stores offer mammoth-sized drinks, from Burger King's 42-ounce "king" offering to 7-Eleven's infamous 44-ounce Super Big Gulp. Americans are free to guzzle down as much as they want, whenever they want—often with free refills!

Few people realize that by doing this they are often loading up on more than 400 calories and consuming more than 100 grams of sugar (not counting refills). There is no denying that mega-expansion of beverage sizes has affected the younger generation. The average teenager now drinks approximately two 12-ounce cans of carbonated soft drinks a day, meaning he or she takes in approximately 20 teaspoons of sugar a day in beverages alone. In 1950 Americans drank four times as much milk as soda; yet today, according to the USDA, that has been reversed, with Americans drinking four times as much soda as milk.[7]

Since soda consumption has replaced milk in many teens' diets, they will likely be at an increased risk of developing osteoporosis, a gradual thinning of bone tissue and loss of bone density. Is it any wonder the CDC reports that over the past three decades the national obesity rate has more than tripled in teenagers?[8] Soda consumption is a huge contributing factor.

The health risks of drinking sodas are obvious. A study published in 2007 in the journal *Circulation* suggests that drinking one or more sodas a day—including diet sodas—is associated with an increase of other risk factors for heart disease. Among those evaluated, those who drank a soda or more each day increased their risk of becoming obese by 31 percent, had a 30 percent higher chance of increasing their waistline, a 25 percent increase in the likelihood of developing elevated blood sugar levels, and were 32 percent more prone to developing lower HDL (good) cholesterol levels. And it made no difference whether it was regular or diet.[9]

As the connection between sodas and obesity continues to solidify, we know one thing for certain: this "liquid candy," which contains approximately 10 percent of the average American's calories in his or her diet, is certainly not all it's cracked up to be.[10]

Alcohol's Girth

After sodas, the most common beverage people consume is alcohol. Like carbonated soft drinks, alcohol poses an obstacle to weight loss. While carbohydrates and proteins have 4 calories per gram, and fat has 9, alcohol comes in around 7 calories per gram. In other words, alcohol is closer in calories to fat than carbohydrates.

Worse, alcohol increases blood sugar levels, leading to elevated insulin levels, which programs the body for weight gain, insulin resistance, and fat storage. Your body will preferentially use alcoholic fuel before it burns stored fat. Worse, alcohol decreases our ability to control our eating while decreasing our inhibitions. So at the same time alcohol stimulates our appetite, it causes us to lose our ability to say no to tempting high-calorie foods.

By far the most widely consumed alcoholic beverage is beer, which is notoriously high in carbohydrates. A typical 12-ounce can contains 148 calories and 13 grams of carbohydrates. While advertisers have helped turn the beer-guzzling, pot-bellied football fan into a cultural icon, obesity and type 2 diabetes fueled by six-packs is no laughing matter. People are "bubble wrapping" their beer bellies with increasing regularity. The omentum is this fatty drape of tissue that hangs beneath the muscles inside the abdomen. This toxic fat is associated with high cholesterol, hypertension, type 2 diabetes, and heart disease.

Typically, the more alcohol you drink, the larger this fatty omentum and the more difficult it is to lose weight. Alcohol alone causes weight gain, but when combined with sugars and stress, your body literally becomes like a belly-fat-forming machine. Some of the worst examples are found during "happy hour" at bars nationwide. After a stress-filled day, many workers like to relieve tension with a social drink. Few recognize that such favorites as a pint-sized margarita contain more than 670 calories and 43 grams of carbohydrates. Coupled with high stress levels, empty stomachs, and handfuls of sweet-and-salty bar snacks, they are creating an epidemic of obesity and type 2 diabetes.

Coffee and Other Caffeinated Beverages

SHOT TO THE HEART

According to the coffee connoisseurs at Italian manufacturer Illy Coffee, a shot of espresso has 35 percent less caffeine than a cup of brewed coffee.[11]

Both alcohol and caffeine act as mild diuretics, which increases urination and water loss. Therefore some people may notice some mild weight loss when consuming alcoholic and caffeinated beverages. What they are losing is only temporary water weight. Many Americans are unknowingly mildly dehydrated, and instead of drinking water that hydrates them, they turn to coffee and other caffeinated beverages, becoming stuck in the caffeine trap

Now, I am not opposed to drinking coffee, which is a good source of antioxidants and can help prevent type 2 diabetes, Parkinson's disease, and

Alzheimer's disease (see next sidebar). However, our national trend toward consuming high-calorie coffee drinks, such as lattes and cappuccinos, is helping fuel the obesity and diabetes epidemics. With a Starbucks on every corner and coffee available at restaurants, supermarkets, and gas stations alike, these drinks are as problematic as sodas. As with carbonated drinks, coffee comes in ever-increasing sizes. When you combine size with the extras ("care for a shot of vanilla syrup or cream with that?") that often go into these drinks, it is easy to see how the line between sodas and coffees is vanishing.

Take the grande Caffe Mocha with whipped cream and 2 percent milk, and you have a whopping 330 calories, 175 milligrams of caffeine, and 35 grams of sugar. The venti Caffe Vanilla Frappuccino Blended Coffee with whipped cream checks in at a mammoth 530 calories, 125 milligrams of caffeine, and 88 grams of sugar.[12]

COFFEE LOWERS RISK OF DEVELOPING DIABETES

Three different studies have shown that coffee consumption helps decrease the risk of developing type 2 diabetes. An analysis of more than seventeen thousand Dutch men and women found that the more coffee a person drinks, the lower the risk for developing type 2 diabetes. Consuming three to four cups of coffee a day decreased the risk of developing diabetes by 23 percent; people who drank over seven cups a day cut their risk in half.[13]

A Finnish study found that consuming three to four cups of coffee a day decreased type 2 diabetes risk by 24 percent, and consuming ten or more cups a day lowered the risk by 61 percent.[14]

Another study of coffee consumption explored the benefits of caffeinated versus decaffeinated coffee. Men who drank one to three cups of decaf coffee a day decreased their risk of diabetes by 9 percent, while those who drank four or more cups a day lowered it by 26 percent.[15]

Please note that these studies pertain to *preventing* diabetes. More studies are needed before we can conclusively state the effects of coffee in people who are already diabetic. Some studies have shown that excessive caffeine raises blood sugar. Unfortunately, most Americans consume coffee loaded with sugar and cream, which is likely to raise blood sugar as well. For this reason I do not advise people with diabetes to drink more than one or two cups of organic coffee per day.

If you are interested in preventing diabetes, an alternative to drinking coffee is taking coffee berry extract. Coffee berry is the fruit that produces coffee beans. The powerful phytonutrients that quench free radicals and help manage blood sugar are found in the whole fruit and not just the bean. I generally recommend 100 milligrams of coffee berry extract, three times a day.

For years many nutritionists have recommended caffeine for weight loss. Caffeine is able to briefly and mildly increase the metabolic rate, making you more alert, energetic, and productive. This usually translates to a more active, calorie-burning lifestyle. Nine out of ten Americans regularly consume some type of caffeine and in moderate doses (150 to 300 milligrams a day), equivalent to about one to two cups of coffee a day.[16] This is not harmful, nor does it cause weight gain. *It is what you add to your coffee that sets you up for weight gain and diabetes.* Especially if you use sugar, artificial sweeteners, or cream. By using liquid stevia, a natural sweetener, and organic skim milk in place of cream, you can dramatically lower caloric intake.

Caffeine also acts as a mild appetite suppressant. It helps stimulate *thermogenesis*, which is how your body generates heat. This helps raise your metabolic rate. Although there is no evidence that increased caffeine intake either causes or prevents significant weight loss, long-term studies have linked higher coffee intake with a lower risk of developing a number of diseases.

However, before you start drinking three or more cups of coffee a day based on this statement, realize that there are side effects. Excessive amounts of caffeine can cause insomnia, a rapid heart rate, and nervous feelings. People may experience headaches from consuming too much caffeine or if they suddenly stop consuming it. Caffeine may also raise one's blood pressure and may trigger an arrhythmia in rare situations. Therefore consult your physician before consuming excess caffeine.

Fruit Juices

I have already exposed the myth that people who switch from regular to diet sodas lose more weight. Ever since the smoothie craze hit, I have encountered numerous people who treat smoothies, fruit drinks, and juices like the new diet soda. Even though such juices as orange, apple, grape, and others have far more vitamins, minerals, antioxidants, and nutrients, they also contain hefty amounts of sugar (especially fructose). Some juices have about the same number of calories and sugar as sodas. Twelve ounces of "healthy" juices can contain approximately 150 calories, or the same calories and sugar as a regular can of Pepsi, Mountain Dew, or A&W Root Beer.

If that weren't bad enough, manufacturers extract fiber—the key ingredient for weight loss and curbing the appetite—from the juice. To make it worse, they usually add additional sugar during processing. Although the standard serving size of fruit juice is only three-fourths of a cup (6 ounces), many Americans consume twice that. Why? They have been mentally programmed to consume soda-can-sized servings of all beverages. Instead of juice, try eating the whole fruit, which is more satisfying and much higher in fiber. However, some diabetics, especially type 1 diabetics and some type 2 diabetics, may even need to avoid most fruits since they may raise their blood sugar.

A word of warning about smoothies: despite their healthy image, they are loaded with sugar. Study the nutrition labels of products in places like Planet Smoothie, Jamba Juice, Smoothie King, or Dunkin Donuts, and you will see that the serving sizes are huge and stuffed with calories. A small (16 ounces) Strawberry Banana Smoothie from Dunkin Donuts packs 360 calories and 69 grams of sugar. Just as bad, a 20-ounce Immune Builder smoothie from Smoothie King, which includes strawberries and bananas, contains 384 calories and 80 grams of sugar. These are just two of the hundreds of combinations available.

> **LIQUIDATION**
>
> Don't depend on your thirst level to determine if you need liquids. During dehydration your thirst mechanism actually shuts off as your hunger increases.[17]

The same warning rings true of many sports drinks, such as Gatorade. While some liquid replenishers have lower calorie and sugar counts than soda and come loaded with electrolytes, vitamins, or both, a 12-ounce bottle of Gatorade's G Series Pro 01 Prime contains 43 grams of sugar and 330 calories.[18] Without the awareness of the calories and sugar in your favorite beverage, you can easily sabotage your weight-loss efforts and tip the scale toward diabetes problems.

Fresh, Pure Water

The best weight-loss beverage is still the world's most natural and abundant: water. Although water makes up approximately two-thirds of our bodies, it is the most important nutrient to consume—more than soda, coffee, beer, or juice. We lose over two quarts a day just through breathing, perspiration, urination, and body wastes.[19] Since we cannot store water in our bodies as a camel, that water must be replaced throughout the day.

Most people need *at least* one to two quarts a day. If you take your weight in pounds and divide by two, you can calculate a more accurate figure. However, if your diet contains adequate amount of fruits and vegetables (five to seven servings a day), those foods will contribute approximately one-half to one-third of your water needs. Instead of eight cups a day you would only need four to six. Adequate water intake is essential to weight loss because water helps fuel your metabolism.

One caution: I am not talking about tap water, which typically contains chlorine, fluoride, and other chemicals. The best kind to help you lose weight is clean, pure filtered or spring water. Otherwise you will contaminate your body with impurities while simultaneously trying to nourish it.

RULE OF THUMB: H_2O

- Drink an 8- to 16-ounce glass immediately after waking up or half an hour before breakfast.
- Drink a glass fifteen to thirty minutes before meals or two hours after (except dinner) (the more you drink, the fuller you will feel).
- With meals, drink only 4 to 8 ounces at room temperature.
- Avoid drinking large quantities after 7:00 p.m.

Many people grew up drinking tap water. Loaded with chlorine, this may taste similar to swimming pool water. I will never forget the childhood vacation when our parents took us to a restaurant that served sodas from a soda machine that used tap water. The "soda" tasted so heavy of chlorine that my sister and I spit it out.

When people say they hate the taste of water, it is usually because they have had lousy water most of their lives and have trained their taste buds with sugary sodas. They often find it hard to wean themselves from these beverages. When patients proclaim their distaste for water, I advise pure spring water or sparkling water with a squeeze of lemon or lime and a few drops of stevia. (For extensive information about types of water, water filters, and sugary coffees, fruit juices, sweet tea, and the like, see *The Seven Pillars of Health* and *Eat This and Live!*)

Tea: The Health Drink

Drinking tea is another great way to supplement water intake. When I visited England several years ago, I fell in love with teatime. Every afternoon we took a break, drinking a cup or two, along with a few bites of cheese and crackers. It left us feeling satisfied for hours. Sadly, most Americans choose afternoon sodas or high-calorie coffee breaks, often supplemented with a doughnut, candy bar, or chips. As I mentioned earlier, only 3.8 percent of total US beverage consumption is tea. That is unfortunate since teas' health benefits are well documented.

Though there are hundreds of teas, the four main groupings are black, green, oolong, and white. Each is highly beneficial health-wise, mainly because of their high content of flavonoids. These flavonoids may help decrease the risk of diabetes, heart disease, and certain cancers, including skin, breast, lung, colon, bladder, ovarian, and esophageal cancers. They assist in blocking oxidation of bad cholesterol (LDL), decrease inflammation, and improve blood vessel function. They also help maintain a normal blood sugar and improve the immune system. In addition, research shows that drinking two cups a day decreases the risk of developing ovarian cancer by nearly 50 percent.[20]

The best news for someone struggling with obesity is that tea—especially green tea—helps to burn fat. Green tea contains a specific catechin phytonutrient called epigallocatechin gallate (EGCG). This substance stimulates the production of norepinephrine, which boosts the metabolic rate. The EGCG in green tea increases the metabolic rate for as long as twenty-four hours and stimulates the body to burn fat. Studies have shown its effectiveness with weight loss, even in those who do not restrict calories.[21]

Green tea also contains an amino acid, L-theanine, that calms and relaxes the body and helps relieve stress. A person typically feels its effects within thirty minutes and feels relaxed for approximately two hours. One study found that drinking five cups of green tea a day was as effective as taking an antidepressant.[22] Water, or green or regular tea with a few drops of liquid stevia, are the beverages I recommend to patients wanting to lose weight.

SEEING RED

Rooibos is an herb used as a tea and is solely grown in the southern tip of South Africa. Red tea has the same antioxidants as green tea but, unlike black tea, doesn't contain tannins, which assist in raising iron levels.

Yerba mate is an herbal infusion that is becoming increasingly popular as more people become aware of its health benefits. While recent headlines have been focused on its weight-loss aspects, for centuries Argentinians have consumed yerba mate as an herbal tonic to reduce fatigue, aid digestion, and boost the immune system.

Yerba mate's antioxidant power exceeds that of green tea, broccoli, and orange juice. The vitamins in mate include A, C, E, B_1, B_2, and B complex; and its minerals include calcium, iron, magnesium, selenium, manganese, phosphates, chlorophyll, hydrochloric acid, pantothenic acid, and choline.[23]

Herbal Infusions

Herbal infusions look like tea; most are packed like teas. However, the herbs are not tea since they do not come from the *Camellia sinensis* bush. They are typically made of barks, such as cinnamon bark; flowers, including chamomile and hibiscus; fruits, such as orange peel; and grasses, such as lemongrass. Herbal infusions with a few drops of stevia are another variety of delicious low-calorie beverages that can help you wean from sodas.

Hunger-Satisfying Beverages and Liquids

Vegetable juices, especially tomato juice or V8 vegetable juice, satisfy hunger much better than other beverages. This is because they stay in the stomach longer, increasing your "full" feeling. They are generally on the low-glycemic end, which makes them a good alternative.

Soups, especially the broth-based (not cream-based) vegetable and bean types, are excellent for weight loss. In fact, many times a soup can be so filling that when you finish it, you are less likely to desire additional food. Soup also takes longer to eat, which helps to satisfy the appetite.

Remember, the problem most Americans have with beverages is that they consume too much of the wrong type. This is a double whammy, packing on additional calories and sugar while stirring up the appetite. In place of sodas and high-calorie coffees, beers, fruit juices, smoothies, and sport drinks, drink more water and teas. You will be amazed at how small changes will program you for weight loss and help you overcome diabetes.

IT ALL BEGINS WITH "WAIST MANAGEMENT"

Chapter 13

YOUR WAIST AND YOUR WEIGHT: POWERFUL KEYS TO REVERSING DIABETES

Have you ever ridden the Kingda Ka at Six Flags in New Jersey? At 456 feet it is taller than the Statue of Liberty. Dropping 418 feet and reaching speeds of 128 miles per hour, the nation's fastest roller coaster promises riders jaw-dropping excitement. Just behind it is northern Ohio's Top Thrill Dragster, which stretches 420 feet into the air and hurtles along at 120 miles per hour. This Cedar Point ride has a cousin: the Millennium Force, dropping 300 feet of its 310-feet height and zipping along at 93 miles per hour. Six Flags Magic Mountain in Valencia, California, reaches 100 miles per hour as it drops 328 feet.[1]

Dieting can be compared to a roller-coaster ride, with one additional feature: instead of ending in a couple minutes, it never lets up and makes life miserable when it jerks you back up the weight-filled mountain. After a while it becomes difficult to find another reason to continue. In nearly three decades of practicing medicine, I have met countless numbers of overweight ex-dieters who were stuck in self-defeating mental attitudes toward weight loss. Their outlook sabotaged any hope of losing pounds.

Have you been battling a weight problem all of your life? No one has to tell you that many cases of diabetes are directly linked to obesity. Determine right now that, with God's help, you will get to your ideal weight and stay there. Perhaps you've been overweight for so long that you've given up. In the back of your mind you may even be thinking, "It's impossible for me to lose weight."

The truth is that your thinking is also your biggest obstacle to weight loss. If you want to lose weight but have been stuck on a dieting roller coaster, you can likely list 101 reasons *not to* diet. Who wants to embark on a boring, rigid, tasteless food regimen? At the same time, though, none of us want to be overweight or obese. Most people want to look good, feel good, and live a diabetes-free, healthy life.

It's Your Life

Take a look at the top ten excuses for not dieting listed below. Do you see the potential for a downward spiral when you get stuck in this kind of thinking? It is a self-propelling trap. Most dieters become virtual excuse-makers, first blaming their circumstances and then themselves for their failures. Most reach a point where they either give in or see a doctor as a last resort.

TOP TEN EXCUSES FOR NOT DIETING

1. "I just can't resist my favorite foods."
2. "My social life is just too crazy."
3. "I don't have time to lose weight or plan meals."
4. "My family and friends won't support me."
5. "I don't have anyone to hold me accountable."
6. "It's too confusing to find which diet works for me."
7. "I travel too much."
8. "Dieting is too restrictive."
9. "It's too expensive to diet."
10. "I'm just too impatient to diet."[2]

The common problem I see among repeat dieters is that they focus on their weight instead of the simple lifestyle and dietary changes they need to make. Then, when their weight doesn't budge, they get discouraged and often stop the program all together. Or there is the other extreme, when people hit their target weight and abandon all reason, quickly sliding back into old eating patterns—the same ones that got them on the diet in the first place!

A Powerful Key to Prevention

Weight control is a powerful key to the reversal and the prevention of diabetes. Type 2 diabetes is directly linked to obesity and diets rich in sugars, refined carbohydrates, and fats. Since it is far better to prevent diabetes altogether rather than to reverse the disease and ask God to heal you afterward, I encourage you to lose weight if you are seeking to prevent diabetes. If you already have type 2 diabetes, weight control is essential.

Why Do You Want to Lose Weight?

It is great to set your mind to something and accept responsibility for your actions, whether looking at the past or toward the future. Yet such a radical shift in perspective can easily become just another mental pep talk that eventually fizzles out. What must accompany this change of heart is an underlying reason—one that comes straight from the heart. To switch to a can-do lifestyle, you need something that compels you from deep within.

Over the years I have observed that if your motive for losing weight is for any person other than yourself, the odds of failure are high. You should be doing this *for yourself*, to make you healthy, not to please someone else. Unfortunately too many women are tempted to lose weight for their spouse or boyfriend. Inevitably these are the women who find themselves back in the blame-shame-guilt cycle, particularly if this other person walks out of their life. I hate to sound cynical, but I have seen too many women do this and gradually regain their weight.

Many obese people are the same way. They have heard plenty of reasons from others why they should lose weight, yet they lack a personal driving force for *why* they should do it. If you are overweight and have never identified this reason, I urge you to do what I suggest to my obese patients: disrobe in front of a full-length mirror at home. Then analyze yourself from the front and back. Ask yourself: What are the main things that concern or bother me about being overweight or obese? Is it:

- The size of your hips, thighs, waist, or buttocks?
- The way your clothes fit?
- The way people treat or mistreat you?
- The embarrassing comments others make about you?
- Rejection from family members, friends, or coworkers?
- Being passed over for promotions because of your weight?
- Because your health is being affected by your weight?
- Because you have type 2 diabetes and do not want to develop the complications of diabetes?

Some people can answer these questions more easily by writing their thoughts in a journal. If that is the case, sit down and take the time to do it. This is an important exercise. If you are completely honest, the answers may change your life. As you come to grips with why you—and only you—want to lose weight and have decided to do so, you are ready to take responsibility for controlling your weight. Most individuals who have lost weight and kept it off did just that. Making this choice empowered them to lose weight by developing new, healthy habits. You may have unique reasons that only come by looking in the mirror, but the important thing is that you arrive in a new place of hope, determination, and purpose.

Facing the Tough Questions

Will weight loss improve your marriage? You would think that the obvious answer is yes. However, after treating many overweight couples, I have often found that is not necessarily true. When one spouse loses weight and the other one does not, many times the spouse who has lost weight gets more attention from the opposite sex at work, out shopping, or while running errands. Some men and women have never had this kind of attention. It is flattering and enticing. Are you and your spouse prepared for possible feelings of jealousy, intimidation, and flattery? At the other extreme, some people have subconsciously gained weight to protect themselves from the pain of being rejected or from going through another painful relationship or breakup. Have you thought through how these issues affect your current and future health?

Also, will you be ready to purchase a new wardrobe in a few months? While the very thought of shopping excites most women, some men get physically ill at the notion of buying expensive new clothing. In addition, are you prepared for the possibility of a promotion or demotion at work? Yes, a leaner and trimmer image may be all you need for that promotion. Or it may spark jealousy from your boss, who reacts by moving you to another department. Understand that by losing weight, people will see you differently and treat you differently.

My point in asking these questions is not to plant fear or worry in your mind but to help you recognize that things will change when you lose weight—often drastically. I want you to be prepared to deal with these changes. Some patients who lose large amounts of weight ultimately need psychological counseling. To me that is a wonderful sign that they are accepting drastic changes and allowing others to help them walk through them. If you feel you need such guidance, don't hesitate to seek it out, maybe even before you start losing. The important thing is that you ask yourself these questions now so that you will not sabotage your weight loss later with wrong thoughts.

Also, examine the issue of timing, which often gets overlooked when people decide to embark on a life-changing journey. Earlier I listed ten common excuses for not dieting, but the truth is you only need one. It is important that you make sure the timing is right for you and that you have counted the cost before you start. Here's a statement that may surprise you: if you are in the midst of a major stressful time in your life such as a divorce, a life-threatening illness, a serious accident, a lawsuit, an IRS audit, a move, a job change, or some other major life event, *it is time to start.*

Before you question my sanity, hear me out. I realize that most diet books would tell you to forgo the diet until the major stress passes. However, it is in the midst of chaos that you want to find a lifestyle that can bring sanity, peace, assurance, and hope. Over the years I have found that when simple dietary and lifestyle principles are practiced regularly, they help you to manage stress and prevent stress eating.

Weight-Gain Mentality

Earlier I stated that your biggest obstacle for weight loss is your thinking. Most of my overweight and obese patients are stuck in what I call weight-gain mentality. They unknowingly have their mental channel tuned to it. As a result they continue to attract more weight to themselves. I tell patients dealing with this problem that their autopilot is stuck on weight gain. You may have seen the same thing happening in your life. It is vital to remember that the ultimate success of any weight-loss program depends not on how much you eat but on what you think and believe.

The Bible repeatedly makes mention of this, often as the law of seedtime and harvest. Galatians 6:7 states, "Whatever a man sows, that he will also reap." In other words, if a farmer plants wheat, he will reap a harvest of wheat; if he plants corn, he will reap a harvest of corn. Elsewhere, Proverbs 23:7 says of a person that "as he thinks in his heart, so is he." This simply means that whatever you think about most, you will eventually become. Similarly, Jesus says in Mark 11:24, "Whatever things you ask when you pray, believe that you receive them, and you will have them."

Since it is important that you believe you can achieve weight loss, it vital to speak affirmations of your desired weight, pants size, or dress size aloud throughout the day. Even if you weigh 250 pounds, you can state aloud that you see yourself weighing 140 pounds or wearing a size 8, or whatever pants or dress size you desire. Hebrews 11:1 defines faith as "the substance of things hoped for, the evidence of things not seen." Romans 4:17 speaks of calling those things that are not as though they are. So if you hope to weigh 140 pounds or wear a size 8 pair of jeans, start visualizing yourself at that weight and speak it aloud a few times a day.

Do not say, "I have to lose 100 pounds," or you will probably always have that many pounds to lose. Likewise, don't get in the habit of saying, "I'm planning on losing 50 pounds," or you will forever be *planning* to do that. Simply look at the picture of you at your desired weight and speak your desired weight aloud: "I see myself weighing _____ pounds" or "I weigh _____ pounds." (Fill in the blank.) Make that affirmation throughout the day, and as you follow through with your weight-loss program, you will naturally be attracted toward that desired weight, size, or image.

I have seen patients who struggled with weight for years do this, and they turned around and told me that losing weight became one of the easiest things they've ever done! I believe you will be making the same statement when you reach your ideal weight. This is not difficult. Start by making the decision to lose weight for yourself and no one else, and understand that you are the only one responsible for being overweight.

Your Waistline Is Your Lifeline

I've said it before, but it bears repeating: your waist measurement is more important than your weight. Just as you need to change the way you look at weight loss, you need a different way to look at nutrition. Ask God to help you achieve this outlook. You will be surprised at the way your thinking about food gradually changes. Although I do want you to weigh yourself on a regular basis, I also want you to start looking at your waistline as a key indicator of diabetes management. This is why the diet for managing and reversing diabetes that I provide in this book is called the Rapid Waist Reduction Diet.

Typically if your waist measurement increases, your blood sugar will increase; if your waist measurement decreases, your blood sugar will decrease. By focusing on your waistline and following a doctor's plan and exercise advice to shrink your waist, you will find that your blood sugar will drop as your waist shrinks.

Let's start by reviewing how to measure your waist. Over the years I've discovered that many men do not do this correctly. They may have a 52-inch waist, but they don't realize it because they can still yank on their old jeans with a 32-inch waist. This is only possible because their huge bellies are overlapping their belts while extended use has stretched the fabric beyond normal limits. Yet they insist they have a 32-inch waist.

BMI, WAIST SIZE, AND TYPE 2 DIABETES

Various health organizations, including the Centers for Disease Control and Prevention (CDC) and the National Institutes of Health (NIH), officially define the terms *overweight* and *obesity* using the body mass index (BMI), which factors in a person's weight relative to height. Most of these organizations define an overweight adult as having a BMI between 25 and 29.9, while an obese adult is anyone with a BMI of 30 or higher.[3] If you would like a chart to help you determine your BMI, refer to my book *The Seven Pillars of Health*. Or do an online search for "BMI" to find tools that can help you calculate yours.

However, an even more important statistic is waist size. The larger your waist, the greater your chances of having type 2 diabetes. For men, waist size is an even better predictor of diabetes than BMI. A thirteen-year study of more than twenty-seven thousand men discovered that:

- A waist size of 34 to 36 inches doubled diabetes risk.
- A waist size of 36 to 38 nearly tripled the risk.
- A waist size of 38 to 40 was associated with five times the risk.
- A waist size of 40 to 62 was associated with twelve times the risk.[4]

In addition, in recent years low-waisted pants became popular in many women's clothing styles. As a result, I have seen more and more women taking their waist measurement way too low.

You should measure your waist around your belly button (and love handles, if you have them). Once I showed them where to measure, I have had patients who were shocked by the reality of their true waist measurement. As reality sinks in, I help them devise the following plan to reach their waist measurement goal.

First, establish a waist measurement goal. Initially the waist measurement goal for a man with diabetes or prediabetes is 40 inches or less. For a woman with prediabetes or diabetes the goal is 35 inches or less.

Second, take your height in inches and divide it by two. Eventually your waist measurement should be equal to this number or less. In other words, your waist should measure half of your height or less. For example, a 5-foot-10-inch man is 70 inches tall, so his waist around the belly button and love handles should be 35 inches or less.

Notice that this is the *second* step, especially for prediabetics and type 2 diabetics. You need to decrease your waist to 40 inches or less (for men) or 35 inches or less (for women) before you worry about reducing it to half your height. Still, I can promise you that with every inch lost in your waist, you will be amazed at the corresponding drop in your blood sugar.

However, sit down and take things a bite at a time as you formulate your own plans to lose weight and reverse the effects of diabetes. The ride may seem all uphill at first, but relax. Over time you will be zipping downhill with the breeze blowing in your face and the frustration of yo-yo diets lost back at the starting line.

Chapter 14

CATCH THE VISION FOR THE NEW YOU

Tim remembered fitting into his favorite suit: the dark blue one his wife had bought for him on their anniversary trip to Paris. It was the same one she asked him to wear when they attended a special banquet or dinner function. A naturally muscular guy from playing sports during his younger years, Tim had always had a hard time finding a suit that fit him just right. Yet this one had. He had to admit that it boosted his confidence every time he wore it.

GASTRIC BANDING SURGERY

As you set your weight-loss goals, you might be thinking of bariatric surgery—gastric bypass, gastric banding, lap bands—as a weight-loss solution. When a person elects this type of surgery, a silicone band is placed around the upper part of the stomach so that it can only hold about an ounce of food. As a result the person feels full faster and eats less. The band can be tightened or loosened, depending on an individual's needs. Most people lose about 40 percent of their excess weight with gastric banding; therefore I believe it can be a viable solution. However, it is not the entire solution. Making healthy choices on a daily basis is the only way to maintain weight loss, even when achieved with the help of surgery. If you opt for gastric banding, remember that you must change your eating habits or you may gain the weight back.

Not anymore, though. Now in his midforties, Tim had not worn this suit for at least eight years. As his gut expanded, his lean, athletic physique faded into the annals of history. He had lost most of his confidence, as I could easily tell when he walked into my office packing 275 pounds on a 5-foot-8-inch frame. Tim had experienced a heart attack the year before and had two coronary artery stents. He suffered from high blood pressure, type 2 diabetes, and excessive cholesterol in his blood, which had forced him onto numerous medications. It didn't take a doctor to see he was the picture of poor health.

I told Tim that if he wanted to decrease his chances of dying early from another heart attack, he needed to lose weight—especially in the abdominal area. His obese, apple-shaped frame held a protruding belly full of toxic fat. Because of it he was at risk for ongoing heart disease, complications of type 2 diabetes, and a host of other diseases. Fortunately my warnings motivated him and his wife, and they made a commitment to losing weight. Still Tim admitted to me that he needed a goal, something he could challenge himself with and strive to meet. He also needed new vision, a belief that he could become as thin as the athlete who once darted down the field to victory.

Visualizing a New You

The same is true for any person hoping for weight-loss success. In the last chapter I mentioned developing the belief that you can achieve this goal. As part of securing yourself in this new place, try performing a simple mental exercise involving visualization. Picture yourself at a healthy weight. What you consistently visualize and confess, you will eventually become.

Close your eyes, and picture yourself walking around in the body that God intended for you to have—the healthy one. You don't have to shop in plus-size stores any longer. You move easily and confidently and no longer huff and puff when you climb stairs. You will wear a bathing suit with comfort and confidence. Are you catching the vision? It is absolutely essential that you see yourself reaching this healthy weight.

As you visualize yourself weighing a certain weight or being a certain size, you will reset your mental autopilot and start to lose weight. Do not say, "I will lose 30 or 40 pounds by faith," or else you will always have 30 or 40 pounds to lose.

To boost your efforts, find a photograph of yourself at or near a healthy or desired weight and place it in different areas of your home, such as on the mirror in your bathroom, on your refrigerator, or as a screensaver on your computers at home and in your office. Some people even tape a copy of the picture to their car's steering wheel or dashboard. Regardless of how many places around the house you want to put your healthy or desired weight photo, it is important to put it in a food journal. As you carry your food journal with you throughout the day and look at the picture, visualize yourself becoming that ideal weight again. Confession is also important, as I discussed in the last chapter; each day confess that, by faith, you weigh your desired weight.

Setting Attainable Goals

Success calls for more than verbal proclamations or wishful thinking, though.

When you are about to embark on a significant lifestyle change to lose a significant amount of weight, it is also crucial to establish attainable goals. I have seen countless people launch into a diet with unrealistic goals. And just as many who dive headfirst into a plan with no set goals in mind. Not surprisingly, both wind up failing. Success requires vision, and when it comes to controlling your weight, that vision must incorporate reality.

An unrealistic goal for weight or clothing size sets you up for discouragement. People who get discouraged will usually quit altogether and eventually regain all the weight. For example, if you are a 5-foot-2-inch female and weigh 300 pounds, you are not likely to be a size 2 or 4 a year from now. You may never get that trim. Realistically, look to be a size 10 or 12 with a waist measurement of 35 inches instead of 45. This is an attainable goal. Once you reach it, you can set another.

Likewise, if you hate going to the gym but have set a goal to work out five days a week for an hour per session, you have just created an unrealistic goal and paved the way to failure. Instead, set a goal of ten thousand steps a day on a pedometer, which simply means more movement or walking. Also, avoid making promises that can be easily broken. For instance, do not tell yourself that you will never have another piece of cake, pie, cookie, or whatever food you crave. Whenever you say that, you have set your autopilot on desiring that food and will most likely want it even more. Instead, as you learn how to develop good eating and discipline habits, avoid using the word *never.*

None of this means that you have to settle for lowered expectations. You can and will look better than you ever have. But the important thing is to first set a goal and then keep it in perspective—both of which can come through taking a few initial measurements.

MEASURING UP

One of the most important keys to losing weight is establishing attainable goals rather than ones that will leave you frustrated, angry, and most likely *gaining* weight. That's why virtually every physician says that when starting a diet, aim for a goal of losing no more than 10 to 15 percent of your total body weight. Once you've reached that, set a new goal—but don't jump the gun. While you can dream big (or in this case small), remember that traveling on the road to weight loss happens one step at a time.

Baby Steps

To help Tim establish his goals, I weighed him on the scale and then measured his waist, hips, body mass index, and body fat percentage. His BMI was more than 40, his body fat checked in at 32 percent, and his hip measurement came in at only 35 inches. However, these were all secondary to what mattered most at that point for Tim: a waist measurement of 46 inches.

As we started down the road to reducing all these numbers, I shared an important warning: weighing yourself daily is one of the worst motivators for weight loss. The first few weeks can seem miraculous as individuals watch the pounds fall off and assume this is all "fat-related" weight. The problem is that many people are losing muscle or water weight, which is guaranteed to lower your metabolic rate and eventually sabotage your weight loss. When you reach the inevitable plateau a few weeks or months later and discouragement sets in, you may give up and quit—all because of focusing too much on a daily or weekly scale reading.

I simply had Tim measure his waist, weight, and body fat percentage once a month—while trying on different pants to gauge his shrinking waistline. It didn't take long for him to line up all his old pairs of pants that he had saved, hoping to one day fit into them again. Most important, of course, was getting back into his favorite suit pants he had worn when he weighed almost 100 pounds less and had a 34-inch waist. Because of that, he originally said he wanted to get down to a weight of 185 pounds and a BMI of 28. Although those

EXPANDING WAISTS

Over the past four decades, the average American male's waist size has gone from 35 inches to 39 (11 percent). Among women, it has increased even more, going from 30 inches to 37 (23 percent). According to the National Institutes of Health, nearly 39 percent of men and 60 percent of women are carrying too much belly fat.[1]

numbers would have technically kept him in the "overweight" category, I explained to him that because of his naturally muscular frame, even those numbers might cause him to lose muscle and subsequently lower his metabolic rate. Instead, the better way was to establish a goal based on his waist measurement. With this in mind, he set his waist measurement goal at 39 inches, which meant he would lose 7 inches of fat from his abdomen.

It's All in the Waist

If you are overweight or obese, I advise you to take the same approach in establishing weight-loss goals. Measure your waistline at your navel or belly button. If you are a man and your waist measurement is 40 inches or more, you are at a much greater risk of heart disease, hypertension, type 2 diabetes, metabolic syndrome, and many other diseases. If you are a woman and your waist measurement is 35 inches or more, you are prone to the same risks. After years of linking only weight and BMI to higher mortality rates and serious illnesses, scientists are understanding—once again—that abdominal fat is a major contributor to the onset of these diseases. Belly fat is highly toxic. After bubble-wrapping itself around internal organs, it secretes powerful inflammatory chemicals that set the stage for type 2 diabetes, heart disease, cancer, and a host of deadly diseases, as well as more weight gain.

That is just one of the reasons your first goal should be to decrease the area holding this toxic fat and keeping you susceptible to disease. After men reduce their waist measurement to 40 inches, their next goal should be to reach 37.5 inches, and eventually their waist measurement goal should be one-half their height in inches or less.

MEASURING TOOLS

Although skin calipers are the easiest devices for measuring body fat percentage, they can also be the most inaccurate. For a more precise (albeit it sometimes expensive) measurement, try:

- Underwater weighing: Fat floats, while lean tissue sinks—making it easy for specialized hydrostatic weighing equipment to get a highly accurate read on how much fat you're actually carrying.

- Dual X-Ray Absorptiometry (DEXA) scan: Using low-level X-rays, this machine takes into consideration your bone mass and muscle mass to calculate your body fat percentage.

- The Bod Pod: A highly accurate (but again expensive) machine that measures how much air you displace.

- Bioelectrical impedance: Less expensive than the other high-tech tools but pricier (and more precise) than a skin caliper, this method measures the speed of an electrical current as it passes through your body. Unfortunately, numerous variables (e.g., full stomach, recent exercise) can sway your results.[2]

Body Fat Percentage

While I see waist size as the most important measurement for establishing weight-loss goals, this does not mean that you can't or shouldn't take other types of measurements—beyond those you can take with a tape measure. Part of the time with patients during their goal-setting stage I spend getting a body fat percentage. I do an initial measurement and then take one a month until they reach their goal.

There are many ways to measure body fat percentage, including a bioimpedance analysis, underwater weighing, and using skinfold calipers. Whatever the method, you need to have your body fat percentage measured the same way each time. Consistency is the key, since the percentage can fluctuate dramatically with inaccurate measurements.

I hold more stock in body fat percentage than I do the body mass index reading. The reason is simple:

accuracy. BMI uses only height and weight to judge how overweight or obese a person is. For example, a twenty-three-year-old professional football player and a fifty-six-year-old executive may both be 5 feet 10 inches tall and weigh 220 pounds. This gives both men a BMI of approximately 35, which is considered obese. In reality, however, the player can have a 32-inch waist and a remarkable 6 percent body fat; the executive can have a 44-inch waist and 33 percent body fat. That is an astounding 27 percent differential in body fat percentage alone, which the BMI doesn't take into account.

Hopefully, you are beginning to see some of the confusion that patients, doctors, and other health-care workers deal with when it comes to varying measurements. Although many physicians simply use BMI to determine if a person is overweight or obese, I strongly believe more accurate assessments come from using body fat percentage and waist measurements.

Rating your body fat percentage

Finding your ideal body fat percentage involves two main factors: sex and age. According to the American Council on Exercise, a body fat percentage greater than 26 percent in men and greater than 32 percent in women is considered obese. A healthy percent body fat in women is 25–31 percent and in men is 18–25 percent. Initially, obese men should aim for a reading of less than 25 percent, while obese women should shoot for less than 32 percent. Eventually aim for a percent body fat in the healthy range.

However, remember that body fat ranks second to your initial focus to reduce your waist measurement. Don't worry; you will find that body fat percentage will naturally decrease along with your waist measurement. Also, women should remember—because of their hormones—that they will have a higher body fat percentage than men. Female hormones cause distribution of fat in the breasts, hips, thighs, and buttocks. A typical woman should have between 7 and 10 percent more body fat than the average man. Many health clubs, nutritionists, and physicians have the equipment to measure your percentage of body fat. Once you have this initial number, log it in your food journal and get it checked each month.

However, don't get too hung up on body fat or other measurements like your BMI reading. Focus on one thing and one thing only: waist measurement. Yes, it's that simple. You really do not need a scale or any other fancy tools—just a tape measure. By focusing on your waist and achieving your goal measurement, you will also lower your blood sugar and may reverse type 2 diabetes.

A Matter of Weight

For some dieters the idea of not looking at a scale every day sounds foreign. Others feel strange if they don't check at least once a week. Yet after helping thousands of individuals lose weight for good, I have seen how most people do better when they either pack up their scale or get rid of it entirely. The reason is almost purely psychological. When dieters lose the wrong type of weight, such as water weight or muscle weight, their skin may sag or wrinkle, their cheeks and eyes may appear hollow, and their muscle mass may melt away. In the meantime, their metabolic rate decreases, their weight plateaus, and they wind up discouraged because each time they hit the scale, the numbers are still the same. Most often these are the people who quit and regain weight.

Don't get me wrong—weight is important. That is why I always get an initial weight for every patient. Still, because of our weight-obsessed culture, the numbers on a scale can easily become the only measure of success. Though tempting to monitor your progress this way, it is not a reliable indicator of fat loss. And losing belly fat should be your primary concern. Avoid the potential depression, guilt, shame, or hopelessness by temporarily putting your scale away.

FIVE "NON-DIGIT" WAYS TO MEASURE WEIGHT LOSS

1. Overall attitude
2. Energy level
3. Fit of clothes
4. Friendly comments and compliments
5. Feeling of taking up less space

Rely more on an old-fashioned tape measure, a pair of old jeans, a food journal, and a monthly body fat percentage measurement while committing to a monthly weigh-in.

Also, weigh yourself on the same day of each month, and make sure you are fully disrobed. If you are a woman, keep in mind that your weight will fluctuate, based on hormonal fluctuations and your menstrual cycle. So do not get discouraged when this occurs.

Once you reach your goal weight, I then recommend that you weigh yourself daily. That is the only time that I recommend this, since this is the best way to maintain your weight loss.

Day by Day

Now that you have your waist measurement goal and have recorded your body measurements, weight, BMI, and body fat percentage (if desired) in your food journal, you don't have to think about these numbers. Your focus should be on taking things one day at a time. Too many people pay so much attention to the final result that they forget to focus on what they are doing day by day. As a result, they battle discouragement along the way.

If you get nothing else from this chapter, understand that losing weight takes time. Plus, everyone is different and loses weight at different rates. Since they typically have more muscle and a higher metabolic rate, men usually lose much faster than women.

This is one reason to avoid weekly weigh-ins; it is too easy to get discouraged if you only lose a half pound in one week or even gain a pound or more because of normal body fluctuations.

Some people gain muscle in the process of losing fat, which often causes their weight loss to go slower. And some individuals are severely metabolically challenged due to chronic dieting, insulin resistance, low thyroid, hormone imbalance, or other factors. This makes each weight-loss experience unique. So don't make the mistake of comparing yourself with someone else who is also trying to lose weight.

You may not be able to control how fast you reach your goal, but you can control how you follow a particular program on a daily basis. When you focus on implementing wise dietary and lifestyle choices day by day, they will eventually become habits. Many experts say that it takes twenty-one days to form a habit. Others think it takes forty; some place it at ninety days. However long it takes, the point is that when you focus on applying principles just for today—without worrying about how you'll face tomorrow or next week—then, over time, it becomes part of your lifestyle. And when that happens, you will find your mind's autopilot set on losing weight. By focusing on one day at a time, you consistently make the right choices. Obviously there will be some exceptional days, such as birthdays, holidays, or anniversaries. You may "cheat" and eat too large a portion of cake or too many high-glycemic foods. Don't let a temporary setback sidetrack you. Remember you are one meal away from getting back on track and again making the right choices.

Success Story

The results that Tim saw show that it is possible to set goals and meet them. He achieved his initial waist measurement of 39 inches—a loss of 7 inches—in just six months. Because he had reached that goal, it gave him the momentum and perseverance to establish another goal. This is often the case with obese people who are able to lose weight, which is why I emphasize setting realistic, attainable goals. Tim's second goal was getting to a waist measurement of 35 inches, which he attained in just four months.

Tim's weight decreased from 275 pounds to 210 pounds in less than a year (and imagine how good that felt). More importantly, he lost 11 inches of waist girth during that time, and his blood sugar levels returned to normal. And his blood pressure and cholesterol also normalized without any medication. He was more active and had more energy at any time since he was young. He combined laser-like vision with realistic goals. In the process, he reversed diabetes and avoided other serious health issues that were sure to follow had he continued down the path of obesity.

Section IV

REVERSING TYPE 2 DIABETES THROUGH DIET

Chapter 15

BEFORE YOU BEGIN THE RAPID WAIST REDUCTION DIET

Still wondering if this book will deliver on the promise to reverse your type 2 diabetes? With the program I now call my Rapid Waist Reduction Diet (RWRD), I have helped countless patients over the years to lose weight as the first step in managing and even reversing their type 2 diabetes. I've seen this program work for them, and I know it can work for you too.

I'm going to outline the program for you in chapters 16 and 17, but first I want you to understand how I came to develop a weight-loss program that can deliver such an amazing promise and also share important information you need to know before proceeding further and embarking on the program.

How the RWRD Program Was Developed

It all actually began over sixty years ago when Dr. A. T. W. Simeons developed a low-calorie diet and worked on his protocol for approximately twenty years. His protocol, *Pounds and Inches*, was published in 1954. When his 500-calorie-a-day, very low-fat and very low-carbohydrate diet was combined with small daily doses of the pregnancy hormone hCG (human chorionic gonadotropin), he claimed it caused the body to release abnormal collections of fat in the problem areas of the hips, thighs, buttocks, waist, and belly.

In Dr. Simeons's day, patients were hospitalized for in-patient treatment for the entire six-week duration of the program. Many consider Dr. Simeons's protocol the best kept medical secret as well as the most effective weight-loss program of all time.

Typically patients on the protocol report having high energy levels, a sense of well-being, and little to no hunger. According to Dr. Simeons, 60 to 70 percent of the patients kept the weight off long-term.

In 2007, consumer advocate Kevin Trudeau made Dr. Simeons's protocol known to the world in his book *The Weight Loss Cure "They" Don't Want You to Know About*. I started recommending the Simeons Protocol and monitoring patients back in 2008. At that time I used hCG injections. However, now I recommend either the sublingual hCG tab that is compounded by a compounding pharmacy or Advanced fat loss drops.* (See Appendix B.) The FDA requires us to inform patients of the following statement: "hCG has not been demonstrated to be an effective adjunctive therapy in the treatment of obesity. There is no substantial evidence that it increases weight loss beyond that resulting from calorie restriction, that it causes a more attractive or 'normal' distribution of fat or that it decreases the hunger and discomfort associated with calorie restricted diets." For women who are still menstruating, I recommend that they start the hCG sublingual tablets when their menstrual period stops; if they are on the protocol for six weeks, they need to go off of the hCG sublingual tablets during their menstrual period.

The first two days of the protocol you need to take the hCG tablets and eat as many good fats and calories as possible, such as salads with lots of organic extra-virgin olive oil, organic peanut butter, almond butter, avocados, hummus, guacamole, seeds, nuts, coconut oil, and other healthy fats. During these two days eat as much fat as you can every three hours.

Results do vary from person to person, but a number of my type 2 diabetic patients have been able to come off all their diabetic medications after following the RWRD and losing belly fat. I have modified the 500 calories in the Simeons Protocol to approximately 1,000 calories in the RWRD, but I've kept Simeons's ratio of proteins, fats, and carbohydrates similar. I have also added more soluble fiber and supplements to boost serotonin levels since low-carbohydrate diets are usually associated with low serotonin levels. Adding soluble fiber also helps with satiety, blood sugar control, and improved bowel movements. This program has been very effective for my type 2 diabetics, and I call it phase one of my Rapid Waist Reduction Diet, which I will outline in chapter 16. Phase one typically lasts four to six weeks and is followed by phase two, which I have outlined in chapter 17.

Make Sure You Can Participate

Certain people cannot participate in the RWRD. Please read the following very carefully and be sure to get the permission of your primary care physician before attempting to follow this protocol. You must be eighteen years of age or older, and certain medical conditions, medications, and supplements may exclude you as a candidate.

---

* As of the printing of this book, the FDA does not allow over-the-counter (OTC) hCG drops to be labeled as homeopathic and make claims about weight loss. It is extremely difficult to get homeopathic hCG drops due to the new FDA regulations. The drops I recommend have been modified to comply with the FDA. The prescription sublingual hCG tabs I recommend also comply with the FDA restrictions as they are a prescribed and not OTC and this new restriction does not pertain to the prescription sublingual hCG drops.

I also want to remind you that if you are prediabetic or diabetic, you must talk to your personal health care practitioner before making any changes to your diet, natural supplements, or medications. The advice in this book is based on general principles of health, but your physician knows your individual situation and needs to be involved to ensure the steps you take to incorporate these principles into your dietary program are done in a way that will work for your particular health needs.

Also, while this is a temporary protocol to help you lose belly fat, it is only the first step in a lifestyle change. The goal of having more than one phase of the diet is to help you stabilize your weight and then return to normal meals that follow healthy eating guidelines. If you are going to manage or even reverse type 2 diabetes, you will have to stick with a healthy way of eating for the long haul. It is the key to keeping this disease at bay and enabling you to live the healthy, abundant life you were designed to live.

In my opinion, by creating two phases of this program, I have combined the best weight-loss program with the best maintenance program. According to Dr. Simeons, his protocol allows your body to maintain its structural fat,

MEDICAL CONDITIONS THAT MAY EXCLUDE YOU FROM THIS PROGRAM

- Pregnant or planning to become pregnant
- Currently breastfeeding
- Surgery—you must be off the RWRD a minimum of two weeks before having surgery. If you have recently had surgery, you must wait a full six weeks before starting the RWRD, and you must inform your surgeon about being on the program prior to surgery.
- Cancer of any kind, except for certain skin cancers
- Heart failure
- Type 1 diabetes—however, people with type 2 diabetes can participate with the consent of a physician since this protocol can possibly reverse their medical condition.
- Chronic renal failure
- Severe anemia
- Epilepsy or any other seizure disorders
- Mental illness including moderate to severe depression, moderate to severe anxiety, suicidal thoughts, ideations, or attempts, bipolar disorder or psychosis

MEDICATIONS THAT MAY EXCLUDE YOU FROM THIS PROGRAM

- Diuretics
- Anti-inflammatory medications
- Coumadin
- Insulin
- Birth control pills—birth control pills will not work with this program.
- All other prescription medications, over-the-counter medications, and nutritional supplements must be cleared by your medical doctor prior to starting the RWRD.

which helps prevent sagging skin and a drawn, tired-looking face. The skin may actually glow and may appear more youthful.

The Diet to End All Diets

I'm not a proponent of dieting. However, because patients I've treated with the RWRD program typically experience consistent, steady weight loss, which keeps them very motivated while they practice incorporating the key dietary and lifestyle components they'll need to manage and reverse their type 2 diabetes, I feel this diet puts an end to all other dieting. My goal is to get you committed to a healthy lifestyle program that will give you the best quality of life possible, and I believe the two phases of this program will result in you no longer being caught in the vicious cycle of yo-yo dieting. I believe the Rapid Waist Reduction Diet is the last diet you will ever need.

As the name reflects, the focus of this program is reducing your waist measurement. Although I have reviewed such topics as calories, fat grams, and glycemic index values, you *won't* track any of these things during phase one or phase two. Instead, during phase one you will learn to select the right type and amount of low-glycemic carbohydrates and combine them with the right amounts of healthy proteins while avoiding most fats. This combination will literally program your body to burn fat, particularly the toxic fat in your belly, which is the key for those suffering from type 2 diabetes. During phase two healthy anti-inflammatory fats will be added in the correct proportions to healthy low-glycemic carbohydrates and healthy proteins.

There are some risks you need to be aware of before you begin.

UNDERSTANDING THE RISKS

In my practice I have patients read the following risks before signing a consent form to begin this program. I believe this information is important for you to know before you agree to participate in the Rapid Waist Reduction Diet.

- I understand the side effects of hCG administration and a low-calorie/nonfat diet can include dizziness, light-headedness, and lowered blood pressure.

- I understand that my blood pressure must be checked at least two times a week.

- I understand that I must be under the care of my primary care physician during the entire cycle of hCG supplementation (four to six weeks).

- I understand that taking diuretics, anti-inflammatory drugs, or Coumadin will require monitoring blood tests, as determined by my physician.

- I understand that there is a limit of 1,000 calories allowed daily on this diet.

- I understand that increasing my caloric intake could alter the results and may increase medical risks.

- I understand that cheating by eating sugary or fatty foods while on phase one can be harmful and may predispose me to forming gallstones.

- I consent to taking sublingual hCG. I agree to be monitored by medical professionals during my weight-loss treatment period. My primary care provider will also monitor any medical condition not related to the RWRD.

- I understand that the FDA has *not* approved hCG for weight loss and that there is no medical data that supports the use of hCG for weight-loss purposes.

- I understand that I will be required to have current (within one month of beginning the RWRD program) lab test results on my chart. These tests are performed to rule out any conditions that could be worsened by the stringent caloric restriction and/or the administration of sublingual hCG in the RWRD program.

- I agree to report any problems or side effects that occur within the time frame of treatment to my medical professionals.

- I understand that I must have an established relationship with a primary care provider before starting this program

- I understand that I must consult with my primary care provider to receive refills on medications that were prescribed by them. Doing so will help minimize confusion between patients and medical providers.

- I understand that the following conditions may prohibit intake of a low-calorie diet:

    - History of recent myocardial infarction (MI)/heart attack
    - History of CVAs and/or TIAs (stroke)
    - Uncontrolled seizures
    - Unstable angina, clotting disorders, or DVT/PE
    - Severe diabetes
    - Severe liver disease (may require a low-protein diet)
    - Severe kidney disease (may require a low-protein diet)
    - Active peptic ulcer disease
    - Active cancers
    - Pregnancy, actively trying to become pregnant, or currently breast-feeding
    - Eating disorder (e.g., anorexia nervosa or bulimia)
    - Severe psychiatric disturbance (e.g., major depression and/or suicide attempts, bipolar disorder, or psychosis)

- ○   Corticosteroid therapy greater than 20 milligrams a day
- ○   Chronic illicit drug usage, addictions, alcoholism, substance abuse

• I understand that failure to comply with protocols—including keeping my primary care physician advised of my medical history, this regimen, and any changes in my condition—may predispose me to develop gallbladder disease, sabotage my weight-loss goals, or cause other harm.

Benefits of Detoxing Before the RWRD

I typically have patients detox for a month prior to phase one to enhance the success of the RWRD program. I believe that preparing your body for the very low-calorie diet and hCG phase of the program is an absolute must.

Your body can harbor a host of unpleasant substances, including, but not limited to, pesticides, herbicides, parasites, candida, and heavy metals. Toxins are stored in the dense fat that will be released during phase one of the RWRD program. If all the toxins from the liver, colon, and fat were released at once, the results could be detrimental to your health.

In addition, most overweight people are actually nutritionally deficient. I have found that ridding the body of toxins, parasites, yeast, and fungus, in addition to restoring it nutritionally, ensures success of the RWRD program. I believe an entire month (thirty days) is needed in order to get your body ready for phase one, so I highly recommend you participate in a thirty-day detox program before beginning the RWRD program. The thirty-day detox diet is simply my candida diet and eating only organic foods. Refer to *The Bible Cure for Candida and Yeast Infections* for more information.

Results vary from one individual to the next, but my patients who have gone through thirty days of detoxification before starting the RWRD program usually report the following benefits:

- Improved mental clarity
- Flatter abdomen
- Decreased appetite and cravings
- Less depressed mood
- Improved energy level
- Feeling of overall vitality and better health
- Weight loss while detoxing
- Acceleration of the rate of weight loss in RWRD phase one

I have carefully determined that taking the following supplements for a month prior to phase one will help detox your body, rid it of parasites and candida, and boost your nutritional status:

- Beta TCP: Two tablets three times a day. This will help support gallbladder function, which usually becomes sluggish with age. (See Appendix B.)

- Divine Health Living Multivitamin: One scoop in the morning. This supplement is loaded with vitamins, minerals, antioxidants, phytonutrients, or Max N-Fuse. (See Appendix B.)

- Divine Health Probiotic: Two capsules in the morning on an empty stomach. This restores beneficial, healthy bacteria to your gastrointestinal tract. (See Appendix B.)

- Divine Health Fiber Formula: One heaping teaspoon in 4 ounces water every night at bedtime. This assists in cleansing the intestines of toxins, and it also aids in regularity of bowel movements. (See Appendix B.)

- Vitamin D_3: 2,000 IUs a day assists the immune system. (See Appendix B.)

- Living Omega: One capsule two times a day. This is pharmaceutical-grade fish oil that supports cardiovascular, brain, joint, and eye health. (See Appendix B.)

- Cellgevity: Two capsules two times a day. This supports liver detoxification and has antioxidant and anti-inflammatory protection. (See Appendix B.)

While on this month-long detox program, I encourage you to eat only organic food if possible to prevent recontamination of toxins in your body. Weight training and brisk aerobic exercise are highly recommended during this thirty-day detox as well, but only mild walking is recommended during phase one of the RWRD. Once you have successfully completed thirty days of detoxing, you are ready for phase one, which is based on a modification of the Simeons Protocol.

Chapter 16

RAPID WAIST REDUCTION
DIET, PHASE ONE

Before starting phase one of the Rapid Waist Reduction Diet, take your photo and record your weight, waist measurement, blood pressure, BMI, and percent of body fat (if available). Make certain your primary care physician monitors your blood pressure if you are taking medication for hypertension. *Your blood pressure usually lowers significantly during treatment.* Here are a few other suggestions you should follow:

- Only take medications (including over-the-counter medications) specified by your primary care physician, who should monitor and adjust dosing as needed.

- Supplements can help with overall health during the protocol, including PGX fiber, Divine Health Fiber Formula, Serotonin Max, Living Multivitamin or Max N-Fuse, and Cellgevity. (See Appendix B.)

- Strictly follow the following list of approved foods. Phase one of the Rapid Waist Reduction Diet is an approximately 1,000-calorie-a-day diet that starts on the third day you begin taking hCG sublingual tablets or the fat loss drops. (See Appendix B.) It needs to be followed exactly.

- Do *not* attempt this diet without the hCG tablets. The slightest variation can prevent weight loss. If you find that the hCG tablets are not enough to curb your appetite, it is fine to take both the fat loss drops and the hCG sublingual tablets at the same time. This should be very effective in controlling your appetite as you stick to the eating plan.

Phase One Eating Guidelines

Dr. Simeons would place his patients on a 500-calorie-a-day diet with injections of hCG and would hospitalize his patients for the entire six-week duration of the program. I have found over the years that the majority of my diabetic patients would not stay on the 500-calorie-a-day diet, nor would they fulfill their commitment to twice-a-week checkups at my office. I then decided to modify his program for my diabetic patients and simply doubled the calorie intake to approximately 1,000 calories a day. Since most of my diabetic patients either skipped breakfast or ate a light breakfast, I added a choice for breakfast of either a meal consisting of meat and vegetables or fruit or a specific type of protein drink.

There are many different foods, especially fruits and vegetables, that have the same calories or even lower calories than the fruits and vegetables listed; however, they interfere with weight loss on the hCG program. This is why it's important that you commit to only eating approved foods. Here are some helpful tips to keep in mind:

- When choosing meats, always choose the leanest cuts of organic meats and trim off all of the fat.

- All of your foods and beverages need to be organic.

- Tea, coffee, and clean pure water and mineral water are the only drinks allowed.

- Drink coffee or tea in any amount (no sugar and only 1 tablespoon of skim milk is allowed every twenty-four hours). To sweeten, stevia is preferred, but saccharin is allowed.

- You should drink at least 2 quarts of water daily. However, you can drink more than that. Good waters include spring water (such as Mountain Valley Spring Water). Your body may retain water when your water intake falls below its normal requirements. This in turn may slow down your weight loss.

- If you feel dizzy or light-headed during this diet, increase your intake of water, and take PGX fiber with each meal.

- The fruit or the melba toast may be eaten between meals instead of with lunch or dinner, but no more than four items listed for lunch and dinner may be eaten at one meal. Take PGX fiber, two capsules with 8–16 ounces of water if you eat the fruit or melba toast between meals.

- You may have a Grissini breadstick and an apple for breakfast or an orange before bedtime, but these must be deducted from your lunch or dinner rations. (Dr. Simeons preferred the Italian breadsticks called Grissini, which may be more satisfying than melba toast.)

- Do not eat your daily ration of two breads and two fruits at the same time. Ingesting too many carbohydrates at one time slows down weight loss. You may not save food from one day to eat the next.

- There is no restriction on the size of one apple.

- Variants for the meat protein: You may occasionally eat 100 grams or 3 ½ ounces of fat-free cottage cheese. (No other cheese is allowed.) You may occasionally eat one whole egg with three egg whites in place of a meat portion.

- All fat must be trimmed from the raw meat before weighing. Only meats listed are permitted.

- If it is not on the list, *do not eat it in any quantity*. Dr. Simeons spent many years developing this program and found that even substituting okra, artichokes, and so on, which, although of equivalent caloric value, did not produce equivalent results. There is no need to reinvent the wheel. There will be plenty of time for creativity when you get to phase two.

- All meat must be broiled or boiled.

- Vegetables must be raw or steamed.

- The juice of one lemon is allowed for all purposes.

- A small amount of salt, pepper, vinegar, mustard powder, garlic, sweet basil, parsley, thyme, marjoram, and so forth may be used as desired for seasoning, but no oil, butter, or dressing.

- All fresh white fish must be low in mercury (catfish, cod, haddock, herring, mullet, sardine, tilapia, tongol tuna, white-fish, whiting).

- A George Foreman grill/steamer would be very helpful.

- You may use salad spritzers, such as Wishbone spritzers, which contain 1 calorie per spray. Use up to five sprays per salad.

- Salads may be spinach, mixed greens, romaine, cabbage, or arugula.

Other Considerations

- *No creams, oils or lotions* should be used on your face, skin, or body during this program. Topically applied hormones should be in gel form (no creams or oils).

- *No cosmetics* other than lipstick, eyebrow pencil, mascara, and powder should be used. You should use one of the many all-mineral powder cosmetics during this time, such as Bare Minerals, for your foundation.

- *No massages:* The use of a far-infrared sauna is encouraged instead.

- *Sunshine:* Try to get at least five to ten minutes of sun every day.

- *Female cycles:* If you are a menstruating female, you cannot use the hCG sublingual tablets during your menstrual period. I have patients stop taking hCG sublingual tablets during their menstrual period; however, patients usually do not need to do this with the homeopathic drops.

- *Pedometer:* Make sure you get mild exercise in every day. Wearing a pedometer will help to ensure you get your ten thousand steps in for the day.

- *Constipation:* If you experience constipation during the diet, use Divine Health Fiber Formula, 1 heaping teaspoon at bedtime with 4 ounces of water. (See Appendix B.)

Repeating Cycles If You Have More Weight to Lose

Cycle one: first round of hCG

- If you have a small amount of belly fat to lose, then do phase one for four weeks. As soon as the toxic belly fat is gone, you will usually begin to feel hungry again. After losing the toxic fat, you need to go to the phase two program.

- If you have more belly fat to lose, then you can follow phase one for about six weeks.

- If you stop losing weight during phase one, then take an apple day, which means eating six Granny Smith apples (no other foods) throughout the day for one day with as much water, tea, or coffee as you like. Do not eat any of the "list foods." The next day simply resume the 1,000-calorie diet. Do not skip your hCG tablets.

Cycle two: another round of hCG, if needed

- If you need another cycle of hCG tablets, then you should begin again after six weeks of being on the phase two program.

Repeated cycles of hCG

- If you need to repeat several cycles of hCG tablets because you still have weight to lose, you need to wait eight weeks before cycle three. If you have more to lose, wait twelve weeks before cycle four. If you need another cycle, wait twenty weeks before cycle five, and wait six months before cycle six.

Approved Foods for Phase One

Start the following diet and continue it for the next four to six weeks, depending on the amount of weight you need to lose. Choose only from the following approved foods for each meal. You should choose different foods for each meal from day to day. A seven-day meal plan follows this list of approved foods. The meal plan is an example you can use to plan out what you will eat a week at a time.

For breakfast you may substitute a protein shake that contains 18 to 25 grams of protein, less than 3 grams of sugar, and less than 2 grams of fat. (See Appendix B.) You may blend the protein with 8 ounces of water, 8 ounces of unsweetened almond milk (found at most health food stores), 4 ounces of So Delicious unsweetened nonfat coconut milk, and 4 ounces of water, or 8 ounces of water with 1 tablespoon of skim milk. You may also blend ½ cup of frozen strawberries. Another breakfast option, only one time a week, is one egg (omega-3 or pasteurized) with two additional egg whites cooked with a small amount of Pam cooking spray or poached (which is preferred). You may accompany the egg and egg whites with melba toast and fruit.

NOTE: You should choose a different meat and vegetable for lunch and dinner on the same day. You may choose to eat your fruit as a midmorning or midafternoon snack.

APPROVED FOODS FOR PHASE ONE				
Beverages	**Lean Meat/ Protein** (grilled or boiled, 3.5 oz., or 100 g; choose one per meal)	**Vegetables** (raw or steamed, 1 cup; choose one per meal)	**Fruits** (choose one per meal)	**Breads**
• Water • Tea • Coffee (See guidelines for allowable sweetener and milk.)	• Lobster • Veal • Beef • Chicken breast • Crab • Fresh white fish • Shrimp • Bison (buffalo) • Elk • Venison (deer) • Egg (you may occasionally have an egg, either hardboiled or scrambled with a small amount of cooking spray.)	• Spinach • Chard • Chicory • Beet greens • Green salad • Tomato • Celery • Fennel • Onions • Red radishes • Cucumbers • Asparagus • Cabbage	• Apple • Granny Smith apple • ½ grapefruit • ½ cup strawberries (You may choose to eat your fruit for a meal or for a snack.)	• 2 Grissini breadsticks (see Appendix B) • 2 slices melba toast

Seven-Day Meal Plan for Phase One

Remember, the first two days of the phase one protocol you need to take the hCG tablets and eat as many good fats and calories as possible, such as salads with lots of organic extra-virgin olive oil, organic peanut butter, almond butter, avocados, hummus, guacamole, seeds, nuts, coconut oil, and other healthy fats. During these two days eat as much fat as you can every three hours. What follows is a seven-day meal plan that begins on day 3. Remember to take PGX fiber before each meal. Also, the majority of women only need the 3.5 ounces of protein, but some women may want more. They can increase their protein portions up to the men's portion.

Day 3

Breakfast
- Fresh white fish (3.5 oz. for women or 6 oz. for men) OR one egg, hard boiled or poached. You can make an omelet using Pam cooking spray, adding onions, tomato, spinach, chicory, and celery, with salt and pepper to taste. Do NOT include cheese or mushrooms.
- 1 apple
- OR protein shake with fruit

Lunch
- Chicken breast (3.5 oz. for women or 6 oz. for men)
- 1 cup spinach or green salad
- 2 Grissini breadsticks or 2 slices melba toast
- ½ cup strawberries or ½ grapefruit

Dinner
- Lean beef, elk, buffalo, veal, or filet mignon (3.5 oz. for women or 6 oz. for men)
- 1 cup green salad or asparagus
- 2 Grissini breadsticks or 2 slices melba toast

Day 4

Breakfast
- 1 egg and 2 extra egg whites
- ½ grapefruit
- OR protein shake with fruit

Lunch
- Fresh white fish (3.5 oz. for women or 6 oz. for men)
- 1 cup cabbage or green salad

- 2 Grissini breadsticks or 2 slices melba toast
- ½ cup strawberries

Dinner
- Crab or shrimp (3.5 oz. for women or 6 oz. for men)
- 1 cup asparagus or green salad
- 2 Grissini breadsticks or 2 slices melba toast

Day 5

Breakfast
- Fresh white fish (3.5 oz. for women or 6 oz. for men) OR one egg, hard boiled or poached. You can make an omelet using Pam cooking spray, adding onions, tomato, spinach, chicory, and celery, with salt and pepper to taste. Do NOT include cheese or mushrooms.
- 1 Granny Smith apple
- OR protein shake with fruit

Lunch
- Chicken breast (3.5 oz. for women or 6 oz. for men)
- 1 cup tomatoes or green salad
- 2 Grissini breadsticks or 2 slices melba toast
- ½ cup strawberries

Dinner
- Deer, elk, veal, or filet mignon (3.5 oz. for women or 6 oz. for men)
- 1 cup spinach or green salad
- 2 Grissini breadsticks or 2 slices melba toast

Day 6

Breakfast
- Fresh white fish (3.5 oz. for women or 6 oz. for men) OR one egg, hard boiled or poached. You can make an omelet using Pam cooking spray, adding onions, tomato, spinach, chicory, and celery, with salt and pepper to taste. Do NOT include cheese or mushrooms.
- ½ grapefruit
- OR protein shake with fruit

Lunch
- Chicken breast (3.5 oz. for women or 6 oz. for men)
- 1 cup romaine salad with up to 5 sprays of Wishbone salad spritzer

- 2 Grissini breadsticks or 2 slices melba toast
- ½ cup strawberries

Dinner
- Filet mignon (3.5 oz. for women or 6 oz. for men)
- 1 cup spinach or green salad
- 2 Grissini breadsticks or 2 slices melba toast

Day 7

Breakfast
- Shrimp (3.5 oz. for women or 6 oz. for men) OR one egg, hard boiled or poached. You can make an omelet using Pam cooking spray, adding onions, tomato, spinach, chicory, and celery, with salt and pepper to taste. Do NOT include cheese or mushrooms.
- 1 apple
- OR protein shake with fruit

Lunch
- Fresh white fish (3.5 oz. for women or 6 oz. for men)
- 1 cup cucumbers or green salad
- 2 Grissini breadsticks or 2 slices melba toast
- ½ grapefruit

Dinner
- Veal, filet mignon, or extra lean hamburger meat (3.5 oz. for women or 6 oz. for men)
- 1 cup mixed greens salad or asparagus
- 2 Grissini breadsticks or 2 slices melba toast

Day 8

Breakfast
- Fresh white fish (3.5 oz. for women or 6 oz. for men) OR one egg, hard boiled or poached. You can make an omelet using Pam cooking spray, adding onions, tomato, spinach, chicory, and celery, with salt and pepper to taste. Do NOT include cheese or mushrooms.
- ½ cup strawberries
- OR protein shake with fruit

Lunch
- Chicken breast (3.5 oz. for women or 6 oz. for men)
- 1 cup green salad

- 2 Grissini breadsticks or 2 slices melba toast
- ½ grapefruit

Dinner
- Crab (3.5 oz. for women or 6 oz. for men)
- 1 cup spinach
- 2 Grissini breadsticks or 2 slices melba toast

Day 9

Breakfast
- 1 hardboiled egg
- ½ cup strawberries

Lunch
- Chicken breast (3.5 oz. for women or 6 oz. for men)
- 1 cup green salad
- 2 Grissini breadsticks or 2 slices melba toast
- 1 Granny Smith apple

Dinner
- Lean beef (3.5 oz. for women or 6 oz. for men)
- 1 cup red radishes or salad
- 2 Grissini breadsticks or 2 slices melba toast

Even though this diet seems restricted, you will be encouraged as you see inches disappear, belly fat melt off, and your blood sugar improve! Stick to it! More food selections will be on the way (in the next phase).

Chapter 17

RAPID WAIST REDUCTION DIET, PHASE TWO

Congratulations! You have completed the toughest phase. Now is the time for you to get creative with your food choices. You may eat any free-range and organic foods you like except for sugars and starches. Starches include potatoes, corn, grains (including breads and pasta), or any food including these choices. Sugars include honey, molasses, maple syrup, corn syrup, lactose (milk), and, of course, sugar.

You will be on this phase for at least six weeks. At the end of these six weeks, if you have more belly fat to lose, then you will need to repeat another hCG cycle (phase one). However, if you have lost most of your belly fat and your blood sugars are normal, you can begin simply following the principles of the anti-inflammatory diet I outlined in chapter 6 or follow the program in my book *Dr. Colbert's "I Can Do This" Diet.*

WHAT TO DO IF YOU AREN'T LOSING WEIGHT

If for some reason you are not achieving optimal results with the RWRD program, you may need one of the following tests. Refer back to the earlier chapters of this book where I discussed the hidden reasons behind some people's inability to lose weight. Talk to your primary care physician or refer to the appendix for information on these tests.

- NeuroScience Adrenal to test your neurotransmitters and adrenal function
- Hormone testing
- ALCAT or Sage food sensitivity testing
- Anxiety/depression testing
- Thyroid hormone testing
- Further metabolic testing
- Yeast/candida testing

Once you move on to the anti-inflammatory diet or the "I Can Do This" diet, make sure you weigh yourself daily. If your weight starts to climb, you will need to repeat this six-week phase two program. If belly fat starts collecting, then you will need to go back on phase one.

I've divided phase two in to two sub-phases. Why? It takes three weeks for your new, lower weight to stabilize. It would be a shame to ruin your hard work by reintroducing sugars and starches too quickly.

Therefore, phase two has a no-carbohydrate stage for three weeks. Beginning with week four, a few healthy carbohydrates such as beans, peas, lentils, oatmeal, and high-fiber cereals are allowed. You can begin using unsweetened almond milk or unsweetened nonfat coconut milk (instead of cow's milk). You don't *have* to add these starches back into your diet in week four; you might find you no longer desire them, which is perfectly fine.

Once a healthy waist size is reached and blood sugars are controlled, you can then follow an anti-inflammatory diet or the "I Can Do This" diet, but you will always need to avoid sugar and desserts. You will also need to weigh yourself daily and go back on phase one or two if you start gaining weight again.

Eating Guidelines for Phase Two

Breakfast

I can't overemphasize that breakfast is the most important meal of the day and a key to weight loss and reversing diabetes. I have already mentioned the importance of fiber and its role in controlling appetite. Getting enough fiber at breakfast is also instrumental to stabilizing your blood sugar for hours, boosting energy, and keeping your mind sharp and your digestive system working optimally. I often call fiber nature's street sweeper for your GI tract.

To control hunger and keep your GI tract functioning optimally during phase two, you should eat 5 to 10 grams of fiber per meal and 3 to 6 grams in a snack, with a mixture of soluble and insoluble fiber. Since most people consume so little fiber, let me also offer a word of caution. Starting with 10 grams of fiber a meal may cause excessive gas and abdominal discomfort. Don't worry—your body will adjust. However, you may need to gradually increase intake by starting with 5 grams and possibly working up to 10. I use fiber supplements with meals and snacks to insure that one is getting adequate fiber, and by taking it before meals, it many times helps control appetite. After avoiding starches for the first three weeks of phase two, you can begin eating unsweetened oatmeal with stevia, Just Like Sugar, or xylitol, which are natural sweeteners.

Lunch and dinner

I've grouped lunch and dinner together because I want to promote a different mind-set, one that grasps that these meals are secondary to breakfast. Although there may be a wider variety of items to choose from for lunch and dinner than there are at breakfast, that is simply because most of our "taste buds" are a little more expansive later in the day. We don't typically wake up craving mahi mahi, asparagus, or sweet potatoes. Don't confuse having more options with thinking you need to eat more at these meals.

Carbs

Remember: no carbs such as pasta, rice, bread, or starchy vegetables for the first three weeks of phase two. This period is carbohydrate free. Starting with week four, you may have beans, peas, and legumes with your meals. However, for all six weeks of phase two you can have as many non-starchy vegetables as desired. You may also sprinkle Butter Buds or Molly McButter on them, or use Smart Balance Butter Burst spray to improve the taste and flavor of your vegetables. Or you can season them with spices.

Proteins

Generally, most meats and fish contain approximately 7 grams of protein per ounce. I recommend 2 to 8 ounces of protein per serving—2 to 6 for women and 3 to 8 for men, depending on lean body mass and activity level.

Some species of fish contain more mercury, PCBs (polychlorinated biphenyls), and other contaminants. Fish that are higher in mercury include shark, swordfish, king mackerel, and tilefish. Albacore tuna and canned tuna contain moderate amounts. Fish low in mercury include haddock, herring, Atlantic mackerel, ocean perch, pollack, salmon (both fresh and canned), sardines, tilapia, trout, and tongol tuna.

Young children, pregnant women, women who may become pregnant, or women who are nursing should avoid eating fish high in mercury. The American College of Obstetricians and Gynecologists recommends a maximum of two 6-ounce servings of fish each week for pregnant women.[1] The American Academy of Pediatrics recommends children and nursing women consume no more than 7 ounces of high-mercury-level fish per week.[2] Realize that all fish increasingly contain more mercury, which is toxic to fetuses and to children's brains. In addition, farm-raised fish are generally prone to containing more PCBs than wild fish.

Fats

It is best to choose salad spritzers that are very, very low in fat. During the rapid waist reduction phase we must restrict fat, as well as grains and most other complex carbohydrates, to the bare minimum in order to burn belly fat. I also recommend the new salad spritzers sold in supermarkets, including Wishbone and Ken's Lite Accents brands. They have only 1 calorie per spray; in my opinion they are superior to other salad dressing options. Nonfat dressings are an option, but most people do not enjoy their taste—and enjoying what you eat is crucial to your success. Most patients enjoy one of the new salad spritzers with only 1 calorie per spray.

Making a Meal

As an example, let's construct either a lunch or dinner using some of the items just listed. To start with a beverage, you can drink a glass of spring, filtered, or sparkling water with a squeeze of lemon or lime. You may also drink tea sweetened with stevia or Just Like Sugar and a squeeze of lemon or lime.

Keep salads healthy

When eating out, skip the bread and start your meal with a salad made of large dark-green leaves and plenty of cucumbers, tomatoes, raw carrots, and onions. You may add brussels sprouts or broccoli spears. Then add ten sprays of a salad spritzer. I believe the easiest way to cut fat is to use a salad spritzer with only minimal fat per spray. Be careful to stick to salad spritzers, since this minimizes your fat intake. Leave off the cheese and croutons.

Most people forget that 10 cups of romaine lettuce only has about 100 calories, while a mere 1 ½ tablespoons of most salad dressings contains an equivalent amount of calories. People hoping to lose weight often get into trouble by eating salads smothered with high-calorie salad dressings. A large Caesar salad may only have 10 calories in the salad leaves but more than 1,000 calories worth of dressing.

Soup is not an option

Next up for your meal is a soup. Select a low-sodium broth-based kind, such as vegetable or bean. These are very filling and will usually prevent you from overeating. Avoid cream-based soups, such as clam chowder or broccoli cheddar, which are high in calories. Make sure your soup is low in sodium (preferably less than 500 milligrams) and low in fat (less than 10 grams). One of the key ingredients for a healthy soup is fiber, so look for those that have at least 3 grams. When it comes to fiber, the higher the better. Finally, don't overdo it on the carbohydrate content. Many soups are loaded with high-glycemic carbs, such as white rice and pasta. Choose vegetable soups, such as minestrone or black bean. Make sure for dinner you choose non-cream-based vegetable soups.

If, by chance, you are still extremely hungry after salad and soup, you can take some fiber capsules. Take two to four PGX fiber capsules—again with 8 to 16 ounces of water. When you do this before you eat your entrée, you fill your stomach faster and are less likely to overeat the wrong types of foods.

Guidelines for entrées

Stick with the guideline mentioned previously of a 2- to 6-ounce serving of protein for women and a 3- to 8-ounce serving for men. Do not deep-fry your meat, but instead stir-fry, bake, broil, grill, steam, or boil it. It's actually healthier to cook the meats at lower temperatures; therefore, steaming, boiling, and stir-frying are healthier methods of cooking. For example, try a grilled chicken breast flavored with low-sodium seasonings. (Watch out for high-carb, high-calorie marinades.) Along with your main source of protein, add a serving of vegetables, such as broccoli, which should take up about half of your plate.

Next, select a low-glycemic starch, such as ½ cup for women and 1 cup for men of beans, peas, lentils, legumes, or sweet potatoes. While women can have one serving and men one and a half to two servings of starch for breakfast and lunch, they should avoid starch and fruit for dinner except for beans, peas, and lentils.

If you are eating out, remember that most entrée serving sizes are double or triple the recommended serving size. Simply eat half the protein and low-glycemic starch and save the rest for another meal or snack. Or ask if you can share with another person at the table.

Save desserts for special occasions

After reaching your goal waist measurement and provided your blood sugar is normal, on very rare occasions you may eat a treat, i.e., dark chocolate or another very small dessert. Prior to enjoying a dessert, I recommend that you take two to four PGX fiber capsules with 8 to 16 ounces of water. This not only lowers the dessert's glycemic index value, but it also helps you feel fuller. With desserts it is especially important to practice mindfulness and savor each bite so that you do not overeat and sabotage weight-loss efforts or cause your blood sugar levels to spike. If you do eat dessert, it's best to eat it for lunch or at an early dinner (before four o'clock) and decrease your starch intake for that meal. Also, take PGX fiber or Divine Health Fiber Formula afterward. (See Appendix B.)

Approved Foods for Phase Two

Low-glycemic, non-grain carbs (three to four servings per day—
breakfast, lunch, and snacks; no carbs after 6:00 p.m. except
non-starchy vegetables or "green carbs," which are unlimited)

Legumes and Beans and Starches Serving = ½ cup (women) and ½ –1 cup (men) (Not allowed for the first three weeks of phase two)	• Beans: kidney, lima, navy, pinto, red, black • Black-eyed peas • Green peas • Butter beans • Chickpeas (garbanzo beans) • Green beans • Lentils • Yams • Sweet potatoes
Cereals (Not allowed for the first three weeks of phase two; cereals must be combined with unsweetened almond milk or unsweetened nonfat coconut milk)	• Old fashioned oatmeal or steel-cut oatmeal (1 serving for women; 1–2 servings for men) • Quaker Oats High-Fiber Instant Oatmeal (plain or cinnamon), 1 packet • Quaker Oat Bran Cereal
Low-Glycemic Fruits ½ cup (Fruit only allowed in the morning)	• Blackberries • Blueberries • Raspberries • ½ grapefruit • Granny Smith apple • Kiwi • Strawberries

Approved Foods for Phase Two (continued)

Low-glycemic, non-grain carbs (three to four servings per day—
breakfast, lunch, and snacks; no carbs after 6:00 p.m. except
non-starchy vegetables or "green carbs," which are unlimited)

Vegetables	
Serving = at least ½ cup or more (women) and 1 cup or more (men). If desired, you may add Butter Buds, Molly McButter, Smart Balance Butter Burst spray, or spices to your vegetables	• Asparagus • Bell peppers • Broccoli • Brussels sprouts • Butternut squash • Cabbage or sauerkraut • Carrots (limit to ½ cup and eat raw) • Cauliflower • Celery • Collard greens • Cucumbers • Eggplant • Lettuce • Okra • Onions • Spinach • Squash • String beans • Taro • Tomato • Turnips • Watercress • Zucchini

Approved Foods for Phase Two (continued)

Lean proteins (limit to every three to four days—at each meal and snack)

Dairy It is best to avoid dairy, but if you must have it, choose nonfat cottage cheese or cream cheese or certain Greek yogurts.	• Cottage cheese, nonfat plain: ½ cup • Cream cheese, fat-free (Philadelphia): 4 tablespoons • Low-fat Greek yogurt, plain or vanilla (must be without fruit, fruit syrup, or honey)
Eggs	• Eggs (pastured or organic preferred): two to three large eggs or one egg yolk with three egg whites
Meats Serving = 2 to 6 ounces for women and 3 to 8 ounces for men, depending on lean body mass and activity level (do not deep-fry meats)	• Beef, extra lean (preferably organic or free-range; remove all visible fats): limit total red meat consumption to less than 18 ounces a week • Buffalo, bison, elk, caribou, venison, goat, ostrich • Chicken and turkey (remove skins) • Turkey bacon • Turkey sausage • Fish (cod, flounder, haddock, herring, halibut, mahi-mahi, sea bass, tilapia, perch, snapper, tongol tuna, orange roughy, salmon, trout, sardines, mackerel): choose wild rather than farm raised • Pork* (lean ham, lean pork chops, pork tenderloin, Canadian bacon): limit pork to one to two servings per week • Shellfish* (shrimp, crab, lobster, scallops, oysters, mussels)

If eating pork or shellfish bothers you for religious reasons, I recommend that you avoid it. However, there is no scientific research to prove that these foods are harmful if you eat moderate amounts of organic, free-range selections.

Approved Foods for Phase Two (continued)

Healthy fats and oils (two servings per day: one serving for breakfast, 1 serving for lunch, and ⅓ serving with each snack, but none for dinner or evening snack)

Fats (May use a small amount of Pam spray)	• Almond butter: 2 tablespoons • Almonds: about 18 almonds (1 ounce) • Organic peanut butter: 2 tablespoons • Peanuts: 1 ounce • Pecans: 1 ounce • Cashews: 1 ounce • Avocado, fresh: ½ cup, pureed • Guacamole: ⅓ cup • Hummus: 8 tablespoons or ½ cup • Smart Balance Butter Burst Spray: 5 sprays • Organic extra-virgin olive oil: 1 tablespoon • Cold-pressed peanut oil: 1 tablespoon • High-oleic sunflower oil: 1 tablespoon • Cold-pressed sesame oil: 1 tablespoon • Cold-pressed avocado oil: 1 tablespoon • High-oleic safflower oil: 1 tablespoon • Pumpkin seeds: 2 tablespoons or 1 ounce • Sunflower seeds: 2 tablespoons or 1 ounce • Flaxseeds: 3 tablespoons or 1 ounce

Approved Foods for Phase Two (continued)	
Salad Dressings Serving = 10 sprays Use only spritzers with 1 calorie per spray; limit to 10 sprays	• Balsamic vinaigrette (Wishbone Salad Spritzers Balsamic Breeze) • Ken's Steakhouse Salad Spritzers
PGX fiber	I recommend two to four PGX fiber capsules with 8 to 16 ounces of water before each meal

It is my mission to help you maintain your weight and enjoy a healthier lifestyle and method of eating. When you achieve your desired waist measurement or weight, you will weigh yourself as soon as you get out of bed and empty your bladder. Weigh without clothes. It is very important for you to take your scales with you when you travel.

Any weight gain greater than 2 pounds over your final phase two weight is significant. If this happens, you need to first follow phase two very strictly, and if your weight doesn't drop, repeat an hCG cycle (phase one) as outlined in chapter 18. Some diabetics will need to stay on phase two permanently to control their blood sugar.

The next lifestyle change that reverses type 2 diabetes involves the incredible benefits of healthy snacking. Once you've moved on to the anti-inflammatory diet or the "I Can Do This" diet, healthy snacking will be an important component of your life. Turn to chapter 18 to learn how the right snacks will help prevent hunger, stabilize your blood glucose levels, and keep type 2 diabetes at bay.

TREATS AND CHEATS

Though many years have passed, I still remember those carefree days of my youth, sitting around a campfire that lit up the pitch-black sky for miles. On these monthly outings with our Scout troop, everyone loved huddling around the fire and staring at its glow while we talked and enjoyed its warmth against the cool night air. Its glow had an unspoken command: if we wanted to continue enjoying the heat, someone had to stoke the fire during the night. I can remember often waking up, shivering, and walking over to the fire to put more wood on it. Every Boy Scout understood that the more wood you put on the fire, the hotter and longer it burned. If we did this throughout the night, we could wake up warm.

Snacks help fuel your body in a similar way. By consuming "mini-meals" in between your three main meals, you stoke your body's metabolic fires, which enable you to burn more calories throughout the day. If it were just a matter of keeping your dietary fires burning, however, many people would not have weight issues. The problem starts with cravings.

Waging War With a Snack

If you are like many people, at some point during the day you probably experience an overwhelming desire for a particular food—usually something you know you should avoid. On the days when you do not feel like fighting the battle, the craving quickly goes from a thought to a single bite to an all-out binge session. If you're like most people struggling with their weight, afterward you feel guilty, ashamed, and maybe even hopeless over the thought that you are locked into a grueling, never-ending struggle with your appetite.

Sound familiar? I encounter this with patients every day. They may be eating three healthy meals a day, getting regular activity, practicing portion control, and avoiding sodas and sweets. Yet without fail, in the midafternoon or post-dinner hours, it is as if someone flips an appetite switch and all they can think about is food—typically the wrong kind.

The truth is that no matter how many carrots or celery sticks you eat, your cravings are not likely to vanish. But before you put down this book and think that there's no point in fighting, understand this: even though you may not be able to eliminate cravings, you can eventually overcome them. The key is controlling them. And one of the most important and effective ways is by snacking.

Snacking Right

Many people do not understand that a good snack can turn off your appetite and can stop the triggers from setting it off in the first place. And though it seems counterintuitive to some, snacking can help you burn more calories in the process. Researchers have determined that snacking on the right amount of healthy foods, in addition to eating three meals a day, boosts the metabolic rate more than if you only eat three meals each day.[1] Snacking stimulates the body to burn more energy. Eating either a meal or a snack every three to four hours will keep hunger in check as well as boost the metabolic rate.

By now I hope you have caught my emphasis on *quantity* and *quality* when it comes to food, including snacks. It does you no good to eat healthy snacks if you consume too many or too much. According to a survey conducted by the Calorie Control Council, one-third of all adults put "snacking too much" as a main reason their weight-loss efforts had failed.[2] I have had to correct many patients who used the power of snacking as an excuse to essentially add a fourth or fifth meal to their daily intake. Even when they chose healthy foods as snacks, they wound up eating massive portions—and the wrong mixture. This obviously defeats the purpose of a weight-loss plan. Avoiding mountain-sized snacks should be a no-brainer.

Likewise, just because you happen to throw the right amount of something on the fire to prevent it from going out does not mean the fire will necessarily burn longer. You have to throw the right kind of fuel on the fire—or the right kind of snack. Twinkies, Krispy Kreme doughnuts, kettle corn popcorn, and high-sugar granola bars don't count. Each of these is similar to putting hay on a fire; it burns up quickly. Eating the wrong kinds of snacks will usually cause you to crave more high-sugar, processed snacks. In other words, when you habitually down a whole pack of Oreo cookies for a "snack," you fill yourself with the wrong fuel and make it likely you will crave that many again. This is why overweight and obese people can often eat their favorite foods and yet never feel satisfied.

Healthy Snacks

So what makes for a healthy snack to ward off these cravings? The word *diet* conjures up images of things like carrots, celery sticks, and broccoli. Although these are healthy foods, they will definitely not satisfy your appetite or hunger. Trying to restrict yourself to this kind of regimen means you may eventually binge on sugary foods and carbohydrates. The best type of snack food is a mini-meal consisting of healthy protein; a high-fiber, low-glycemic carbohydrate or starch; and some good fat. When mixed together, this food fuel or fuel mixture is digested slowly, causing glucose to trickle into your bloodstream, which controls your hunger for hours.

> **FIVE SNACK DUDS**
>
> 1. Cookies (even if they're fat free, watch out for those calories and sugar)
> 2. Granola bars (some pass the test, but most are loaded with sugar)
> 3. Chips and nachos (fat, fat, fat... the bad kind too)
> 4. Cakes and pastries (tons of calories, lots of sugar and fat, and zero nutrition)
> 5. Crackers (although few are OK, many are loaded with butter or oil)

Portion control is a key to wise snacking. Select half a serving of either a low-glycemic starch or one serving size of fruit. Then add 1 to 2 ounces of a protein and a third of a serving size of fat. Typically this mini-meal should amount to just 100 to 150 calories for women and 150 to 250 calories for men. Here are a few examples of well-rounded snacks.

Morning or afternoon snack

- A piece of fruit (fruit can be eaten whole or blended into kefir); 6 ounces of coconut, low-fat plain kefir, or Greek yogurt; 5 to 10 nuts; and 1 scoop of vanilla or chocolate protein powder

- 2 tablespoons of guacamole with raw carrots or celery and 1 to 2 ounces of turkey, chicken, or roast beef (meat optional)

- 2 tablespoons of hummus with raw carrots or celery (4 inches in diameter) and 1 to 2 ounces of sliced chicken or turkey (meat optional)

- 1 to 2 wedges of Laughing Cow Light cheese and 1 to 2 ounces (for men), 1 ounce for women of smoked salmon or tongol tuna (meat optional)

- Half a cup of nonfat cottage cheese, a piece of low-glycemic fruit (such as a Granny Smith apple), and 5 to 10 nuts

- A small salad with a 1 to 2 ounces of sliced turkey and 2 tablespoons of avocado; use a salad spritzer (meat optional)

- A bowl of broth-based vegetable or bean soup with 1 to 2 ounces of boiled chicken

- Carrots or celery, 1 teaspoon almond butter or peanut butter, and ¼ cup of nonfat cottage cheese

- A protein smoothie made from protein powder (1–2 scoops) mixed with 8 ounces of low-fat coconut milk or coconut kefir or almond milk (option: dilute the coconut milk or kefir or almond milk by reducing it to 4 ounces and combining with 4 ounces of filtered water or spring water)

BAR NONE

Countless dieters go wrong by assuming a snack bar is healthy just because the words health, protein, or low-carb appear on the wrapper. In fact, finding a tasty, healthy, balanced snack bar is a challenge. Most are either loaded with sugars and carbohydrates or with fats—and should be classified as cookies. Others are loaded with low-quality proteins but have no healthy ratio of complex carbohydrates, good fats, and fiber. In addition, many use soy for protein, which is not the best for weight loss. Very few have adequate fiber; most leave you craving more. So you end up eating two, three, or the whole box to satisfy your craving.

Unfortunately, no perfect snack bar exists. The three I recommend, only on occasion but not every day, are the Jay Robb JayBar, any FitSmart bar, and the Nutiva Hemp Chocolate Bar (www.drcolbert.com). The best snack option is still a mini-meal using real food rather than a man-made substitute. However, keep a healthy snack bar in your purse or briefcase for emergencies. Most of these snack bars can be found in health food stores instead of supermarkets. Avoid snack bars sold in most supermarkets—they are high in sugar and refined carbs. Remember, as with every meal, a good fuel ratio for a snack bar is 40 percent low-glycemic carbs, 30 percent healthy fats, and 30 percent quality proteins, along with 3 to 5 grams of fiber per bar.

Be sure to take two PGX fiber capsules with an 8- to 16-ounce glass of water with your snack. And remember you can add as many non-starchy vegetables as you want. To top it off, I recommend a cup of green or black tea, using natural stevia as a sweetener.

Evening snacks

- Protein drink
- Lettuce wraps
- Salad with lean meat
- Vegetable soup with lean meat

A Healthy Snack Stash

I have already urged you to clean out all the junk food, chips, crackers, candies, cookies, ice cream, sodas, and high-sugar beverages from your refrigerator, freezer, pantry, and cabinets. The second part of that equation is keeping these places stocked with healthy snacks, including plenty of low-glycemic fruits, seeds, nuts, hummus, low-fat cheese, avocados, baby carrots, celery, and the like. Get a large bowl and fill it with fruits, especially high-fiber fruits such as Granny Smith apples, kiwi, grapefruit, and all types of berries. Keep different deli meats, such as nitrite-free free-range turkey, chicken, lean roast beef, lean ham, and organic nitrite-free beef jerky, in the refrigerator. I also recommend always having a supply of almond milk or low-fat coconut milk; nonfat, low-fat, or part-skim cheese, such as Laughing Cow Light cheese; nonfat cottage cheese or nonfat cream cheese; nonfat or low-fat plain or vanilla Greek yogurt; and kefir and coconut kefir. All of these are simple items that you can take on the go.

> **GOOD FRUITS**
>
> A Brazilian study found that women who ate three small apples or pears a day lost more weight on a low-calorie diet than those who didn't add fruit to their diet. Because of the high fiber in these fruits, those fruit-eating females also ate fewer calories.[3]

In addition, buy different nut butters, including almond butter and organic peanut butter. Have a supply of hummus, avocado, guacamole, seeds and nuts, tomatoes, and cucumbers readily available so you can mix these with different salads and salad spritzers. (Most salads now come in ready-to-serve bags.) For those who often face time restrictions, you can also have a stash of healthy snack bars mentioned earlier in this chapter. Keep green, black, or white tea; stevia; and a supply of lemons and limes around as well.

Along with making sure you stock your home with these easy snack items, be prepared at work and other places. I tell my female patients to always carry a healthy snack in their purses, such as a Hemp Chocolate Bar, a small bag of nuts, a Granny Smith apple, baby carrots in a resealable plastic bag, and PGX fiber capsules. Keep items that are not perishable in your desk drawer at work. Always be prepared by having plenty of healthy snacks at home, in the office, and on the road. Don't forget: it is important to get snacks that you truly enjoy. Otherwise you won't bother.

Controlling Severe Carb and Sugar Cravings

I have already discussed how our digestive system uses up sugary foods and processed carbohydrates within a couple of hours. This rapid digestion causes appetite triggers to repeatedly fire, raising your blood sugar and insulin levels and ultimately causing you to store fat and gain weight. Even obese people have a natural sense for this process; they know firsthand how quickly a sugar high fades away, only to be met by another irresistible craving for more.

Yet what do you do if your cravings for these high-sugar, starchy items continue? What happens when the different snacks I listed above do not turn off your tremendous cravings for these foods? This is usually the case for those who have low serotonin levels in the brain. Serotonin is an important neurotransmitter that calms us down, helps us control our appetite, and gives us an overall feeling of well-being. Having a low serotonin level causes us to crave sugary foods, chocolates, carbohydrates, and starches.

For many individuals this is a serious matter, not just an occasional hankering for a chocolate bar. These people typically have been under long-term chronic stress and have probably had high cortisol levels for years. They may be chronic low-carb dieters, or they battle insomnia, depression, or PMS. Some may also be compulsive eaters and bingers. They typically think about food all the time and are emotional eaters who use food as comfort whenever they feel lonely, bored, sad, anxious, or angry. Women are more prone to fall in this category than men because the female brain produces 50 percent less serotonin than the male brain.[4] This is also why women often go through "carbohydrate withdrawals" more often. A duo of scientists researched this physiological need for serotonin in some people and identified the problem. Judy Wurtman, PhD, and her husband, Dr. Richard Wurtman—both neuroscientists at the Massachusetts Institute of Technology—discovered that, among other things, there were carbohydrate snacks that could boost serotonin levels in the brain.[5] These could ultimately decrease cravings and help control the appetite. However, diabetics should avoid high-glycemic carbohydrates since they usually elevate the blood sugar and prevent weight loss. I recommend 5-hydroxytryptophan (5-HTP) or Serotonin Max for sugar- and starch-craving patients if they have some of the symptoms of low serotonin levels mentioned above. I usually recommend 50 milligrams of 5-HTP one to three times a day or at bedtime. If you are on an antidepressant medicine, consult your doctor before taking 5-HTP or Serotonin Max. (See Appendix B.)

Serotonin-Boosting Snacks

Once you find the snack that works best for you, I recommend that you put the snack in a resealable plastic bag. Then carry the bag in your car, purse, or briefcase. By eating this snack at the specified times, you will help control your appetite and boost your metabolic rate. I also recommend drinking 8 to 16 ounces of water and taking two to three PGX fiber capsules before eating a snack. Whether you deal with low serotonin levels or not, snacks are a powerful thing for any successful weight-loss program. They help control the appetite, which is one of the strongest forces that can come against your efforts to lose pounds and keep them off. In cases of low brain serotonin levels, this force can seem overwhelming. Let me assure you, it is not. With simple preparation you will soon learn it can be easily managed—even to the point of becoming routine.

Chapter 19

TIPS FOR EATING OUT AND GROCERY SHOPPING

The National Restaurant Association estimates Americans spend 49 percent of their food budget at restaurants. It's no wonder that for 2011 the association forecast the industry would reach a record $604 billion in sales and achieve positive growth after a three-year-long downturn.[1] Clearly, eating out is a way of life for millions of American families. Snapshots of families enjoying home-cooked meals over the dinner table in the 1950s and 1960s have faded into history. Today's occur at places like Burger King, Subway, or McDonald's. The ones taken at home are most likely of everyone gathered around a take-out box.

With America's fast-paced lifestyle, many parents feel they do not have time to prepare family meals, leading to an unhealthy reliance on fast-food restaurants. Meanwhile, singles or couples without children at home have discovered that eating out regularly is easier and may be more economical. Still, there are ways to avoid settling into a convenience-food rut. All of us will eat out from time to time—it is part of modern life. However, if you hope to control your weight, there are basic principles you must understand when deciding what dishes to order at restaurants and which foods to cook at home. The key, in both cases, is knowing how to make wise, healthy choices.

The Twin Culprits

There are two main reasons why eating out sabotages weight-loss efforts. The first is simple: most restaurants serve unhealthy foods. Restaurant owners know that flavor sells. To get repeat customers and generate word-of-mouth, they accentuate flavor through unhealthy cooking. It's the principle of supply-and-demand: the public demands tasty, high-calorie, high-fat, high-sodium meals—and that's what they get. To add insult to injury, these meals are usually loaded with inflammatory fats, sugars, salt, and high-glycemic carbohydrates. And they are low in fiber, fruits, vegetables, and nutritional value. Individuals who consistently eat at such restaurants struggle to shed any weight.

Don't buy the hype, either. Reacting to health advocates and headlines about obesity problems, in the summer of 2011 the restaurant association announced its "Kids LiveWell" initiative. Introduced at nineteen chains, among its criteria are offering a children's meal of 600 calories or less and other items with limited calories, fat, sugars, and sodium, and a serving of fruit, vegetables, or other sensible options.[2] While it is admirable that some restaurants are responding to the obesity crisis, don't think that means you can eat anything on their menus.

In addition, recognize that you can count calories all day long at other meals, but if you continue to dine out regularly without learning healthy habits, your weight-loss efforts *will* fail. It will be like training to compete in the Olympics but showing up for the trials without a clue of how to run a specific event. Unless you come prepared each time you set foot in a restaurant, you will repeatedly blow your chances.

The second reason eating out can sabotage weight loss is huge portion sizes. In chapter 14 I reviewed ever-expanding restaurant portions. Simply put, high-calorie foods plus out-of-control portion sizes equal weight gain and obesity—the equation our culture generally follows.

You can be different by learning to dine out but not succumb to the feasts that tempt you. This starts with understanding portion sizes. Since most servings are large enough to satisfy two people, my wife and I usually share entrées while ordering a side salad and extra vegetables. The majority of restaurants are willing to bring our food on separate plates. If you and your partner cannot agree on an entrée, order separately and ask your server to put half the portion in a to-go box before bringing the food to the table.

Walking Through a Restaurant Meal

Many weight-loss patients ask for advice on ordering the right dishes. When I ask about what they usually eat, I often discover they are making wise choices. Most understand they need to apply the principles I mentioned previously—dividing their plate as they do at home and being mindful of eating a proper mix of foods.

However, what I also learn is they either forget about smaller portions or overlook all the extras they consume. For the sake of simplicity, let's walk through a typical dinner so you get an idea of how to apply wise principles to restaurant meals.

The first question every server asks is, "What would you like to drink?" Don't automatically reply Pepsi, Coke, or sweet tea. You can save hundreds of calories by avoiding sugar-laden sodas or sweet tea, which are liquid candy. Alcohol is another questionable choice. When consumed before or early in your meal, it rapidly enters your bloodstream and can affect judgment and food selections. You are more likely to overeat or be lax about eating unhealthy foods.

This is not to say you can never enjoy a glass of regular (not dessert) wine. Just make sure you drink it with your entrée and limit yourself to one glass. If you are a tea drinker, order unsweetened tea with a wedge of lemon or lime, and carry stevia in your purse or wallet. Sparkling water or bottled water is another excellent choice. Take two to four PGX fiber capsules with 16 ounces of unsweetened tea or water.

After you order a drink, ask your server to bring bread with the entrées, or better yet, refuse the bread all together. Your first temptation is usually bread and butter. Who among us hasn't tried to alleviate hunger pangs by going through three small loaves of bread spread with butter or dipped in olive oil before the salad even hits the table? Also, if you want an appetizer, choose one with vegetables and meats such as a shrimp cocktail. Avoid any that are deep-fried, high in starch and fats (i.e., quesadillas or corn bread), or bread based. Again, it's best to avoid most appetizers.

Remember to order your salad with the dressing on the side and with no croutons, cheese, or fattening side items. It's best to bring your own salad dressing spritzer. Add a bowl of broth-based vegetable or bean soup to fill yourself up before the entrée.

The entrée is your most important dietary decision. Meat, fish, or poultry should be baked, broiled, grilled, or stir-fried in a minimum amount of oil. Avoid anything deep-fried or pan-fried. Always ask if your meat selection will be fried; if so, ask if it can be cooked another way. If the menu does not list a meat serving's ounces, ask your server. If more than 6 ounces (for women) or 8 ounces (for men), ask the server to put at least half in a to-go box. Naturally, you should avoid or significantly limit sauces, cheeses, or gravies. If you must have them, ask that the chef put them in a small side dish. Also, request that vegetables be steamed (unless you prefer them raw) *without* any butter or oils.

There is usually an ample supply of starches—which is why most eating establishments' calorie counts are sky-high. Keep in mind the low-glycemic rule, and don't ruin a balanced meal by indulging in butters or fatty oils. If you're a potato fan, remember that baked potatoes are high glycemic. Instead, choose a sweet potato if possible—and keep it to the size of a tennis ball. When facing limited options, take two to four PGX fiber capsules or drink a glass of water mixed with fiber to lower the starch's glycemic value.

The final (and greatest) temptation is dessert. Be prepared; servers aren't doing their job unless they try to entice you with a tray crammed with mouth-watering treats. The more desserts they sell, the higher the tab and the larger the tip. How to avoid this? Before the meal ends, ask the server to not bring out the dessert tray. If you don't, you will be confronted with a sales presentation trying to persuade you that the double-fudge chocolate sundae with whipped cream *just can't be* that bad.

If you still choose a dessert, avoid downing the dish solo. Share it, and only take a few bites. Savor those bites. After all, your taste buds aren't asking for a mound of dessert—they just want some flavor.

Careful Planning

One of the easiest ways to avoid disaster is preparation, which helps avoid unhealthy foods and overeating. The first rule of thumb: never go out to eat when you feel ravenous. I guarantee that you will eat too much of the wrong foods. Before leaving home, eat a large Granny Smith apple or a healthy snack, such as a Nutiva Hemp Bar. This will pre-fill your stomach and help prevent overeating. You can also drink 16 ounces of water or unsweetened tea and take two to four PGX fiber capsules.

In addition, plan what and where you will eat *before* leaving. When people don't know where they're going and arrive at whatever restaurant they stumble across, they usually have no idea what they will order. If you hope to lose weight, these are bad moves. I suggest patients also plan an early dinner, usually between five and six o'clock. By doing this, they will usually not have to wait for a table (helping to avoid a grumbling stomach) and will finish early enough to burn off some calories before going to bed.

If you know you will spend time with friends or family at a restaurant, plan on practicing mindful eating. Share an entrée with your spouse. Slow down while eating, and chew every bite thoroughly, putting your fork down between bites. All these "little" things go a long way in controlling hunger and weight. Not only will your brain get the message sooner that you are satisfied, but also you will be able to relax and enjoy conversation with loved ones.

Choices of Restaurants

We all have our favorite types of restaurants. Unfortunately, most of us developed those preferences long before we considered healthy eating. For some that is not a problem, since their favorite serves healthy dishes. For others, it may present a challenge. Regardless of preference, it is important to know how to make healthy menu selections. Here's how.

Fast-food restaurants

I link the rise of obesity in our nation with the emergence of fast-food restaurants. Their most popular choices are high in fats, salts, high-glycemic carbohydrates, and calories, and the sodas are loaded with sugar. Not only do fast-food restaurants "supersized" portions trigger weight gain, their processed ingredients ensure that people get caught in a cycle of junk-food cravings. Have you ever wondered why most fast-food restaurants have rock-hard plastic seats? The seats, colors, lighting, air, and other factors are designed to get you to eat in a hurry, leave, and make room for other customers. Then, when you're hungry again in a few hours, they hope you will return.

In the event you can't avoid them, try the following at a typical hamburger-oriented chain: Instead of ordering a double cheeseburger (around 500 calories), large french fries (500 calories), and a large soda (about 300 calories), try a grilled chicken sandwich or a small hamburger. Throw away the top and bottom bun, and squeeze your burger between two napkins to remove excess grease. Cut the hamburger in half and then place both halves of the meat between two lettuce leafs. Instead of mayonnaise and ketchup, choose mustard, tomato, onions, and pickle. Now you have a much healthier burger without excessive high-glycemic carbohydrates and excessive fats.

You can also order a small salad and ask for fat-free dressing (or use just a small portion of a regular packet). For a drink, order unsweetened iced tea or a bottle of water. Instead of french fries, order a baked potato when available, using only one pat of butter or 2 teaspoons of sour cream.

If you eat at a sub shop, imitate Jared Fogle, the Subway guy who lost more than 240 pounds by making the right choices. Choose turkey, lean roast beef, and chicken instead of bologna, pastrami, salami, corned beef, or other fatty selections. Choose a 6-inch sub on the smaller bottom of the bun and not the top portion. Use plenty of vegetables, and top with vinegar; avoid or go easy on the oil. It's best to further cut calories by ordering it in a lettuce or pita wrap.

At fast-food chicken restaurants, instead of fried, choose rotisserie or baked chicken. Peel off the skin and pat the chicken dry with a napkin. Drain the liquid from the coleslaw, and do not eat the biscuit or potatoes.

If you're craving pizza, go easy; it is one of the worst weight-loss saboteurs. Before diving into a slice, eat a large salad. Then have only one slice of pizza, sticking to thin or flatbread crust. Choose chunky tomatoes and other veggies as toppings. Avoid pepperoni and other highly processed meat toppings, and ask for half the cheese (the same way many ask for double cheese). Finally, use a napkin to remove excess oils from the cheese.

Buffet-style restaurants

If you hope to lose weight, it is wise to avoid buffet-style restaurants. Most are loaded with fried foods, unhealthy starches, and an assortment of fattening desserts. They offer too much food and too few wise choices, with the exception of some salads and vegetables.

There are a few alternatives for the all-you-can-eat variety, such as a healthier Sunday buffet at a sit-down restaurant. Many offer beautiful salads, fruits, vegetables, smoked salmon, lean meats, fish, and grilled or baked chicken. Just watch out for high-calorie foods, including desserts. Still, they typically have enough healthy options. Start with a large salad (but go easy on the dressing or use a spritzer) and fruit, followed by an entrée with plenty of vegetables. If you get a dessert, limit yourself to a couple bites, or choose berries and leave off the whipped cream.

Steak houses

These are common choices for special occasions. The portion sizes are so large (including football-sized baked potatoes) that two people can share one entrée. Remember to avoid indulging in the bread beforehand, and choose a lean, petite fillet, grilled or baked chicken, grilled fish, or shellfish. Choose steamed vegetables and a large salad (again, with dressing on the side or in a spritzer). While a shrimp cocktail on occasion is fine, beware of béarnaise sauce, hollandaise sauce, gravies, creamed vegetables, cheese sauce, and au gratin dishes. All are loaded with fat.

Italian restaurants

Even at my favorite restaurants, I have to watch out for eating too much pasta and indulging in high-fat, creamy sauces. I advise starting with a soup—minestrone, pasta fagioli, or broth-based tomato—and a large salad. Limit bread and olive oil, which has 120 calories per tablespoon. Good entrée options include grilled chicken, fish, shellfish, veal, and steak. Avoid fried or Parmesan dishes, such as chicken or veal Parmesan. Ask for your vegetables to be steamed, and avoid the pasta or have it cooked al dente. Don't overdo it on the pasta; the amount should be about the size of a tennis ball. Avoid fat-filled creamy sauces, cheese, and pesto sauce.

Mexican restaurants

Mexican food is usually loaded with fat and starches, starting with the tortilla chips. Since these deep-fried treats are full of calories, ask your server to remove them from the table. Instead, tortilla soup without the chips and black bean soup are good appetizers. In addition, be wary of entrées smothered in melted cheese, which automatically increases the fat count.

Despite these hazards, I enjoy Mexican food, usually choosing fajitas with chicken. You can also get beef or shrimp, and the meat is usually stir-fried or grilled, meaning it is healthier. Add such ingredients as salsa, onions, lettuce, beans, and guacamole. Beware of overeating cheese and sour cream—avoid them if possible, since restaurants rarely serve nonfat varieties.

As for beans, choose red or black but not refried, since they are high in fat. Avoid the rice. If a salad is available, enjoy a large one before your entrée. Avoid the tortilla, and make your fajita with lettuce wraps.

Chinese, Thai, or Vietnamese restaurants

These are usually good choices, provided your meat or seafood is baked, steamed, poached, or stir-fried. Steaming is usually the healthiest method. Some Chinese restaurants stir-fry their meat in excessive oil, using as much as a half a cup. Instead of fried rice or fried noodles, choose brown rice. Remember that eating white rice is similar to eating sugar, based on the glycemic index. Sometimes restaurants will allow you to substitute a serving of rice with vegetables. If not possible, take two to four PGX fiber capsules, and don't eat more than a tennis-ball-sized serving of rice. Avoid sweet and sour, batter-fried, or twice-cooked food (which is high in fat and calories) and oily sauces (i.e., duck). For an appetizer, you can choose wonton or egg drop soup instead of deep-fried egg rolls.

The downside to many Chinese restaurants is that many use monosodium glutamate (MSG) to enhance the flavors of main dishes. I recommend finding one that doesn't use MSG or is willing to not use it on your dishes. MSG has numerous potential reactions. The most common is stimulating your appetite, causing you to become hungry again in a couple hours. More importantly, MSG can lead to severe headaches, heart palpitations, and shortness of breath. (For more information on MSG, refer to my book *The Seven Pillars of Health*.)

Japanese restaurants

Japanese food is usually low in fat and features many vegetables. Unfortunately, it is also high in sodium, primarily because of abundant use of soy sauce. An easy solution to this is to add only a small amount of additional soy sauce (if any) to your food. Sushi is fine; some restaurants prepare it with brown rice. Steamed vegetables, vegetable soups, and salads with dressing on the side are also good choices. Seafood, chicken, and beef can be cooked teriyaki style. Fish can be steamed or poached. Be cautious with eating too much rice, and avoid fried foods.

Indian restaurants

Many Indian foods contain large portions of ghee (clarified butter) or oil, so it's best to find a restaurant willing to limit the amount they use on your dish. Tandoori-cooked (roasted) or grilled fish, chicken, beef, and shrimp are good choices. Avoid deep-fried foods and limit sauces, such as marsala sauce and curry sauce, which are high in fat. If you must have them, get them in a small side dish. Also, it's best to avoid the breads—a major element of Indian food. If you have any, however, choose bread that is baked *nan* instead of the fried *chapatis* bread.

French restaurants

Although French cooking is usually high in fat, most French restaurants serve smaller portions than standard restaurants. In recent years a new type of French cooking, called nouvelle cuisine, has emerged that is generally lower in fat. Whichever style you choose, select meats or fish that are grilled, steamed, or broiled. Avoid foods baked in cheese or creamy sauces, or have the sauces served in side dishes and eat sparingly. Most French restaurants serve an abundance of vegetables and fruit; make them the majority of your meal. Because these restaurants are renowned for their pastries and desserts, it's best to avoid them or to be mindful if you sample a dessert. Savor a few bites and share the remainder.

Family-style restaurants

Foods at these restaurants are typically high in fats; the main courses are often fried. The vegetables are usually loaded with gravy, butter, or oil. Good choices include baked or grilled chicken, turkey, or beef with steamed vegetables. Vegetable soup and a salad (dressing on the side) also make good choices. Avoid the large dinner rolls and butter and fried side dishes. Choose beans, such as lima, pinto, or string beans. If you must have gravy, get it on the side and eat it sparingly. Though raised on Southern cooking, I have learned I can enjoy the foods without all the gravies and fried options.

Grocery Shopping Tips

Now that you have learned more about making wise restaurant choices, you need information about healthy shopping. Many of my patients start eating programs on the wrong foot. They sabotage early weight-loss efforts by stocking their refrigerators, freezers, and pantries with refined, processed, sugary, and fatty foods.

As with restaurants, shopping in grocery stores takes advance planning to avoid common marketing traps. Like restaurants, supermarkets are carefully designed to entice you to buy certain foods—and lots. The cardinal rule is simple: *eat before you shop*. If you arrive hungry, you will be too likely to grab too many comfort foods.

It is no coincidence that when you walk into a grocery store you get hit by the aroma of freshly baked pastries, pies, and cookies. If the slightest bit hungry, your resolve will quickly dissolve. It isn't just you, either. Every decision at the grocery store affects everyone in your family. You can shape your children's future simply by what you stock at home.

Every trip should start at home by making a list of only the items you need. This makes you less prone to impulse purchases. Try to list exact brands and amounts; if confronted with a sale price for a high-calorie, high-fat alternative, you will be more likely to stand your ground.

Perimeter Shopping

Let's start our trip by looking at what's on the perimeter. The healthiest food choices are usually located on the outer aisles. This is where you want to start filling your cart with smart buys.

Fruits and vegetables

As I explained earlier, half of your plate at lunch and dinner should consist of vegetables. You will want to spend an adequate amount of time in this section to choose a variety of vegetables and low-glycemic fruits. Unfortunately, most people always buy the same fruits and vegetables and rarely try anything different. If trying to lose weight, you will likely be eating more vegetables than in the past, so I challenge you to try new things. In the process you may discover a favorite new vegetable or fruit.

My wife, Mary, purchases prepackaged organic vegetables and salads, which can cut preparation time in half. Besides eating them raw, Mary and I often steam, stir-fry, or grill our vegetables. To enhance their flavor, we add spices, seasonings, or such condiments as Molly McButter or Butter Buds. Both of these alternatives are fat and cholesterol free and low in calories (5 calories a teaspoon).

As you're shopping, choose a variety of colors of fruits and vegetables. Each color offers unique, protective phytonutrients and antioxidants. Phytonutrients play a significant role in preventing various cancers and heart disease. Because there are literally thousands—all have tremendous health benefits—I urge people to try to eat all the colors of the rainbow each day.

Remember farmers' markets too. These are seeing a resurgence, thanks to younger people wanting fresh, organic, and locally grown produce. In the United States, most food you find on a grocery store shelf has traveled an average of more than fifteen hundred

FROZEN FRUITS AND VEGETABLES

According to the FDA, frozen fruits and vegetables provide the same nutrients and health benefits as fresh fruits and vegetables.[4]

miles from the farm that produced it.[3] Farmers' markets offer an alternative to long-distance shipping and are located nationwide. Often they offer a wider variety of produce.

Another great source is community-supported agriculture (CSA). This allows you to buy organic produce directly from local farmers. CSAs create a sense of community by connecting farmers and consumers, in addition to establishing a mutually supportive relationship and an economically stable farming operation. You can find more information at www.nal.usda.gov/afsic/pubs/csa/csa.shtml.

Meats and fish

Still on the perimeter, meats are usually found at the back. Always choose lean cuts; I advise free-range, range-fed, organic, or drug- and hormone-free meat and poultry. Most cattle are grain fed, which means fattier meat. Ask the butcher to trim off all visible fat. You can also purchase lean roast beef at the deli.

Since most luncheon meats are fatty, high in sodium, and contain nitrites and nitrates, which form cancer-causing nitrosamines, look for low-sodium, low-fat, and nitrite- and nitrate-free luncheon meats. Chicken and turkey are good choices that you can purchase as luncheon meats or entire portions free of nitrites and nitrates. Chicken strips make good fajitas or in a stir-fry dish.

Wild salmon, sardines, grouper, and tilapia make great seafood choices. Choose wild fish instead of farm-raised fish, since the latter typically have higher levels of chemicals, including PCBs and heavy metals. Although tuna has moderate amounts of mercury, small tuna or tongol tuna is generally low in mercury and available in many health food stores. You may eat shellfish (shrimp, crab, lobsters, and oysters) occasionally, but make sure it is cooked well.

You can also eat lean pork (ham, pork chops, roast, or tenderloin) occasionally. However, make sure the butcher trims off visible fat. Avoid sausage because of its high fat content. While bacon is high in saturated fat, certain nitrite-free turkey bacon is acceptable (and delicious). You may also choose Cornish hens, veal, lamb, duck, bison, or elk—all typically low in fat.

Dairy

With the exception of those allergic to dairy or who are lactose intolerant, most people enjoy dairy. However, not all dairy is healthy. If available, always opt for organic. If too expensive, you can choose regular fat-free or low-fat items. I recommend organic low-fat or fat-free plain kefir or yogurt, as well as small amounts of low-fat or fat-free milk and cheese. But do not eat dairy daily, but instead rotate eating small amounts every three to four days. Other wise choices include fat-free cottage cheese, ricotta cheese, part-skim milk cheese, and Laughing Cow Light. Choose organic butter over regular, but use it sparingly; it is still high in fat. Even though most patients aren't allergic to dairy, many are sensitive to it.

If you experience nasal congestion from eating dairy foods, eliminate all dairy for six weeks, then rotate small amounts of dairy every three to four days. If that doesn't help, try low-fat or nonfat goat milk products instead. Use caution with dairy, and do not get in the habit of eating it every day.

You're Getting Colder

Next comes the frozen foods section. If fresh vegetables are unavailable, choose frozen. Since they are frozen at their ideal ripeness, these chilled veggies may contain more nutrients and antioxidants than fresh—especially those transported across the country, a process that can cause them to lose nutrients.

Frozen dinners

According to the US Bureau of Labor Statistics, the average American household spends nearly $79 annually on frozen meals, or more than they spend on eggs, apples, bananas, oranges, lettuce, or tomatoes. No wonder the frozen food industry nets $3.8 billion a year.[5] The average family cooks and eats a frozen meal about six times a month.[6] For these and other reasons, frozen dinners take up more shelf space than any other type of frozen food. I prefer my patients eating fresh food instead of frozen dinners. The key is finding tasty selections that satisfy but are still healthy and do not sabotage weight loss.

One of the most important factors in finding a good product is learning how to read the nutrition label. Many light frozen dinners contain less than 300 calories, 8 grams of fat or less, and are not filling for most people (especially men). Yet dinners that are more filling are often overflowing with fat and sodium. This is just another reason to avoid most frozen dinners.

Criteria for choosing a healthy frozen dinner

- Men can consume up to 550 calories, while women should aim for 250 to 400. (Most men can choose two low-calorie items if they are each 275 calories or less.)

- Choose meals with less than 15 grams of fat and less than 7.5 grams of saturated fats. Make sure that they contain no trans, hydrogenated, or partially hydrogenated fats.

- Choose meals with 600 milligrams or less of sodium.

- Look for at least 3 grams of fiber; 5 to 10 is preferred. You may supplement this with fiber capsules or fiber powder to reach 5 to 10 grams.

- It should have around 40 grams of carbohydrates or less.

- It should contain at least 15 grams of protein.

- It should contain less than 15 grams of total sugars, including corn syrup and malt dextrin.

I know these guidelines can seem overwhelming, but it is important to make healthy choices by reading nutrition facts on the label. Many people choose low-calorie frozen dinners that meet various criteria but do not satisfy their hunger. That is why it is good to augment frozen dinners with a large salad and some steamed vegetables or a bowl of broth-based vegetable or bean soup.

Some of my favorites are certified organic dinners from Helen's Kitchen. Other good choices include Healthy Choice, Kashi, South Beach Living, Lean Cuisine, or Smart Ones. Below is a sampling:

Healthy Choice
- Traditional Turkey Breast With Gravy and Dressing—300 calories, 550 mg sodium, 4 g fat, 42 g carbs, 21 g protein, 6 g fiber
- Sesame Chicken—230 calories, 600 mg sodium, 6 g fat, 35 g carbs, 12 g protein, 3 g fiber
- Rosemary Chicken With Sweet Potatoes—180 calories, 500 mg sodium, 2.5 g fat, 26 g carbs, 12 g protein, 5 g fiber
- Roasted Chicken Verde—230 calories, 500 mg sodium, 3.5 g fat, 35 g carbs, 14 g protein, 3 g fiber
- Honey Balsamic Chicken—220 calories, 540 mg sodium, 3.5 g fat, 34 g carbs, 12 g protein, 5 g fiber
- Portabello Parmesan Risotto—220 calories, 590 mg sodium, 4 g fat, 35 g carbs, 9 g protein, 4 g fiber

Kashi
- Chicken Pasta Pomodoro—280 calories, 470 mg sodium, 6 g fat, 38 g carbs, 19 g protein, 6 g fiber

Lean Cuisine
- Chicken Florentine Lasagna—290 calories, 650 mg sodium, 6 g fat, 37 g carbs, 21 g protein, 3 g fiber

Smart Ones (Weight Watchers)
- Picante Chicken and Pasta—260 calories, 480 mg sodium, 4 g fat, 32 g carbs, 23 g protein, 4 g fiber

Most frozen dinners—even some listed above—do not contain the perfect fuel mixture for weight loss since they are usually higher in carbohydrates and sugar content and low in protein. Therefore, don't eat them for every meal or even once a day. Limit them to one or two times per week.

Caution: Entering the Inner Aisles

You need to exercise caution when entering the inner aisles of grocery stores. Many products are enticing and attractively packaged yet loaded with sugars, fats, and calories. Here you will find processed foods, junk foods, and countless tempting high-calorie synthetic foods.

Cereals

Choose old-fashioned oatmeal, steel-cut oatmeal, or high-fiber instant oatmeal without sugar or honey. Add some berries, cook them in the oatmeal, and sweeten with stevia or xylitol. I have found that by eliminating most grains, especially wheat and corn, most patients will start losing belly fat. Eating oatmeal every four days is acceptable, except during phase one and the first three weeks of phase two.

Pastas and rice

Avoid pasta and rice for the most part to lose belly fat, but eventually when the blood sugar is controlled, small amounts of brown rice and pasta al dente are allowable.

Breads

It is best to avoid bread to lose belly fat, but Ezekiel 4:9 or sprouted bread may be rarely eaten once every four days, but not during phase one or the first three weeks of phase two. It tastes better if toasted.

Oils

My favorite oil is extra-virgin olive oil and other monounsaturated fats including avocados, almonds, cashews, hazelnuts, pecans, macadamia nuts, peanuts, sunflower seeds, pumpkin seeds, and nut butters. Also, flaxseeds and flaxseed oil are other favorites since they are anti-inflammatory omega-3 fats. So are wild salmon, sardines, and anchovies. If you choose others, make sure they are cold-expeller pressed vegetable or nut oils such as extra-virgin olive oil and high-oleic safflower and sunflower oil. However, even healthy oils are still loaded with calories—approximately 120 calories per tablespoon. Go easy on the oil.

You now have completed most of your grocery shopping and should have avoided purchasing many foods that sabotage weight-loss efforts. Your pantry and refrigerator will now contain the foods that will satisfy your appetite and enable you to lose weight.

Section V

OTHER IMPORTANT STEPS IN REVERSING TYPE 2 DIABETES

Chapter 20

SUPPLEMENTS TO REVERSE DIABETES

The use of multivitamins, minerals, and herbs is rising; adults using some kind of dietary supplement increased from 42 percent in 1988 to 53 percent by 2006. In some cases, this was undoubtedly an attempt to compensate for a poor diet. Says Dr. Orly Avitzur, a medical advisor to *Consumer Reports*, "It's a Band-Aid approach to think you can eat poorly and just take a vitamin and you'll be equal to another person who eats well and exercises and takes care of their health and gets regular checkups. There's no substitute for a healthy lifestyle."[1]

I can't quibble with this observation. Supplements cannot take the place of a complete program to control and reverse type 2 diabetes, which includes weight reduction and especially waist reduction, proper diet, regular physical activity, stress reduction, and hormone replacement therapy. However, once you have adjusted to a healthy eating plan, you can add nutrients and supplements to your diet to help control blood sugar in a systematic, natural way. Such supplements can help those suffering from type 1 or type 2 diabetes; however, type 1 diabetics will *always* need insulin.

Following is a complete list of nutrients and supplements that help fight type 2 diabetes. (If you have type 1 diabetes, these supplements are still helpful to your overall health. However, the ones listed that will be of greatest benefit are alpha lipoic acid, vitamin D, chromium, PGX fiber, omega-3 fats, and supplements for decreasing glycation.)

A Good Multivitamin

A comprehensive multivitamin forms the foundation of a good supplement program. Adequate doses of nutrients found in a comprehensive multivitamin include magnesium, vanadium, biotin, and B vitamins, plus macro minerals and trace minerals. To review some of these:

- Magnesium is essential for glucose balance and is important for the release of insulin and maintenance of the pancreatic beta cells, which produce insulin. Magnesium also increases the affinity and number of insulin receptors, which are on the surface of cells. The recommended daily allowance for magnesium is 350 milligrams a day for men and 280 milligrams a day for women.

- Vanadium is another mineral that assists in the metabolism of glucose.

- Biotin is a B vitamin that helps prevent insulin resistance.

In addition to a multivitamin, you need other nutrients and larger doses of certain vitamins and minerals. Most physicians are unaware of the nutritional supplements that effectively lower blood sugar. You will need to make your doctor aware that you are taking supplements for diabetes. The supplements alone are able to lower your blood sugar significantly, and diabetic medication dosages will eventually need to be lowered accordingly, especially when combined with weight loss, proper diet, and regular activity.

Vitamin D$_3$

Many Americans do not get enough vitamin D$_3$; a close link is developing between a vitamin D$_3$ deficiency and diabetes. A 2009 article by researchers from Loyola University's Marcella Niehoff School of Nursing concluded that an adequate intake of vitamin D may prevent or delay the onset of diabetes and decrease complications for those who are diagnosed with diabetes. Researchers substantiated the role of vitamin D in the prevention and management of glucose intolerance and diabetes.[2]

Vitamin D$_3$ also plays an important role in the secretion of insulin and helping you prevent insulin resistance. Vitamin D$_3$ decreases your blood sugar and increases your body's sensitivity to insulin, thus making the insulin more effective.

I determine vitamin D$_3$ levels in patients by checking their 25-OHD3 level, which measures its level in the blood. I typically try to get the patient's vitamin D$_3$ level to an optimal level of 50 ng/ml to 100 ng/ml. I start most patients on 2,000 IU of vitamin D a day. I may increase that to 4,000 or even 10,000 IU as I monitor their 25-OHD3 level until their vitamin D$_3$ is in the optimal range of 50–100 ng/ml. I then place them on a maintenance dose. A normal vitamin D$_3$ level is greater than 32 ng/ml; however, it is important for diabetics to get their vitamin D level in the optimal range to reap the most benefits from vitamin D$_3$.

Chromium

Chromium is a mineral that is essential for good health. It has long been of interest to diabetes researchers because it is required for normal metabolism of sugar, carbs, protein, and fat. I call chromium "insulin's little helper." Without adequate chromium, insulin cannot function properly.

How much do you need? In 1989 the National Academy of Sciences recommended a daily intake range of chromium for adults and adolescents of 50 to 200 micrograms.[3] The Food and Nutrition Board of the Institute of Medicine has since narrowed this range down to 35 micrograms for men and 25 micrograms for women between the ages of nineteen and fifty.[4]

A well-balanced diet should always be your first step in getting adequate amounts of vitamins, minerals, and other nutrients. However, fewer and fewer foods are providing the needed dietary intake of this important mineral. Whole grains and mushrooms may contain trace amounts, but only if these foods are grown in soils containing chromium. Likewise, seafood and some meats contain chromium, but only if the animals ingested foods containing chromium. Brewer's yeast is the only natural food source high in chromium; however, few people eat this regularly.

Ironically, the standard American diet, which is full of refined sugars and carbohydrates, actually *depletes* your body of chromium since these foods require chromium for metabolism. In addition to avoiding foods

SELECTED FOOD SOURCES OF CHROMIUM

A well-balanced diet does provide you with some chromium; however, the methods used for growing and manufacturing certain foods greatly affect their chromium levels and make it difficult to determine specific amounts of chromium you receive from each food. The following chart shows approximate chromium levels in foods, but it should only be used as a general guide.[5]

FOOD	CHROMIUM (MCG)
Broccoli, 1/2 cup	11
Grape juice, 1 cup	8
English muffin, whole wheat, 1	4
Potatoes, mashed, 1 cup	3
Garlic, dried, 1 teaspoon	3
Basil, dried, 1 tablespoon	2
Beef cubes, 3 ounces	2
Orange juice, 1 cup	2
Turkey breast, 3 ounces	2
Whole-wheat bread, 2 slices	2
Red wine, 5 ounces	1–13
Apple, unpeeled, 1 medium	1
Banana, 1 medium	1
Green beans, 1/2 cup	1
Brewer's yeast, 2 Tbsp.	140 percent of RDA of 20-35 mcg for most adults

high in refined sugars and carbs, consider taking a chromium supplement. Type 2 diabetics in particular tend to be deficient in chromium, which usually aggravates their condition.

Richard A. Anderson, PhD, chief chemist at the USDA Nutrient Requirements and Functions Laboratory, has conducted many studies on chromium supplementation and its effects on diabetes. He says, "Increased intake of chromium has been shown to lead to improvements in glucose, insulin, lipids, and related variables."[6] Be aware that chromium is commonly included in multivitamins, usually in smaller amounts; for example, Centrum Silver only contains 45 micrograms of chromium. For many people this may provide adequate supplementation.[7] Always inform your doctor before making any changes to your diet or supplement program.

There are several forms of chromium used for supplementation, but the most common is chromium picolinate. For type 2 diabetic patients, I typically recommend between 200 and 1,000 micrograms a day of chromium picolinate, taken in divided doses.

One study Dr. Anderson conducted found that type 2 diabetics who consumed 1,000 micrograms per day of chromium improved insulin sensitivity without significant changes in body fat. Type 1 diabetics were able to reduce their insulin dosage by 30 percent after only ten days of taking 200 micrograms of chromium picolinate a day.[8]

Other studies in which researchers gave chromium to people with type 1 and type 2 diabetes have yielded mixed results. However, Dr. Anderson says that studies that show no beneficial effects from chromium for diabetes were usually for those using doses of chromium of 200 micrograms or less, which is inadequate for many diabetics—especially if the chromium is in the form that is poorly absorbed.[9]

The question this poses: Can you take too much chromium? According to Dr. Anderson's research, no discernible toxicity has been found in rats that consumed levels up to several thousand times the dietary reference for chromium for humans (based on body weight). He also says there have not been any documented toxic effects in any of the human studies involving supplemental chromium.[10] Still, do not take massive amounts of any supplement without the advice of your doctor. (See Appendix B.)

Alpha Lipoic Acid

Alpha lipoic acid is an important nutrient for type 1 and type 2 diabetics. Diabetics are more prone to oxidative stress and free radical formation than nondiabetics. Lipoic acid is an amazing antioxidant that works in both water-soluble and fat-soluble compartments of the body and regenerates vitamin C, vitamin E, coenzyme Q_{10}, and glutathione. Lipoic acid also improves insulin resistance in overweight adults suffering from type 2 diabetes.

Lipoic acid can also help relieve several components of metabolic syndrome. It can decrease insulin resistance, improve the lipid profile by decreasing oxidation of LDL cholesterol, and promote weight loss. Lipoic acid has been used in Europe for decades to treat diabetic neuropathy with impressive results.

I usually start diabetic patients on 300 milligrams of alpha lipoic acid twice a day while monitoring their blood sugars. Occasionally I may increase this to 600 milligrams two to three times a day. Some patients develop GI side effects, skin allergies, or decreased thyroid function, so I monitor them closely. Scientific studies using daily doses ranging from 300 milligrams to 1,800 milligrams infer that the most important form of lipoic acid is R-dihydro-lipoic acid, which is the most readily available form.[11] However, for diabetic patients I find that alpha lipoic acid usually works well and is usually less expensive. (See Appendix B.)

Cinnamon

The Chinese have used cinnamon medicinally for more than four thousand years. Ancient Egyptians and Romans also recognized its many uses, and it remains one of the world's most common spices. In recent years cinnamon's therapeutic effects have made headlines. Some research has shown that cinnamon may have insulin-like effects and cause blood sugar to be stored in the form of glycogen. It also contains excellent antioxidant properties.

The most commonly cited study on the effects of cinnamon on diabetics was published in *Diabetes Care* in 2003. Sixty people with type 2 diabetes were divided into six groups of ten patients each. Groups one through three were treated with 1, 3, or 6 grams of cinnamon per day; groups four through six received a placebo. After forty days, the cinnamon groups' reduction in blood sugar was amazing. Their fasting blood sugars decreased by 18 to 29 percent. The placebo group showed no change.[12]

However, whole cinnamon contains oils that may trigger allergic reactions, which is why I recommend a cinnamon extract. One form is Cinnulin PF, which contains the active component found in whole cinnamon without the toxins. USDA studies have indicated that cinnamon extract promotes glucose metabolism and healthy cholesterol levels in people with type 2 diabetes.[13] Cinnamon extract also appears to help glucose transport mechanisms by increasing the insulin signaling pathways. I generally recommend taking 250 milligrams of Cinnulin PF, twice a day. (See Appendix B.)

Omega-3 Fatty Acids

These are simply polyunsaturated fats that come from such foods as fish, fish oil, vegetable oils (especially flaxseed), walnuts, and wheat germ. However, the most beneficial omega-3 fats are fish oils containing EPA and DHA.

Omega-3 fats generally decrease inflammation, lower triglyceride levels, and may help prevent insulin resistance and improve glucose tolerance. Fish oil also helps to decrease the rate of developing diabetic vascular complications. Omega-3 fats also help to reduce the risk of heart disease and stroke and slow the progression of atherosclerosis.

While fish oils are probably the most protective fats for our blood vessels, trans fats are the worst for our blood vessels and can greatly increase one's risk of developing diabetes. Trans fats are hydrogenated fats or partially hydrogenated fats and are ubiquitous in processed foods, fast food, and many choices in restaurants, whether chains or locally owned. One 2009 study showed that only a 2 percent increase in calories from trans fat raised the risk of diabetes in females by 39 percent, and a 5 percent increase in polyunsaturated fats decreased the risk of diabetes by 37 percent.[14]

Dietary fats that are considered beneficial include flaxseeds, fish oils, and monounsaturated fats, including avocados, extra-virgin olive oil, almond butter, macadamia nuts, peanuts, sunflower seeds, pumpkin seeds, and nut butters. I only recommend one type of omega-6 fats, which is GLA. GLA is present in borage oil, black currant seed oil, and evening primrose oil. (See chapter 11 and *Dr. Colbert's "I Can Do This" Diet* for more information on fats.)

However, a word of caution is needed with fish oils, since some supplements may contain mercury, pesticides, or PCBs. I usually place my patients with prediabetes and those with diabetes on 320 to 1,000 milligrams of fish oils three times a day. If they have high triglyceride levels, I may increase the daily dose to 4,000 to 5,000 milligrams. (See Appendix B.)

Supplements to Decrease Glycation

Carnosine

Glycation is the name for protein molecules that bind to glucose molecules and form advanced glycation end-products (AGEs). Glycated proteins produce fifty times more free radicals than nonglycated proteins. Typical manifestations of this are skin wrinkling and brain degeneration, as well as most of the long-term complications of diabetes. Both prediabetics and diabetics are much more prone to glycation and, as a result, will age prematurely.

The amino acid carnosine, however, helps stabilize and protect cell membranes from glycation. Carnosine is a safe and effective nutrient for inhibiting glycation. I usually recommend at least 1,000 milligrams a day of carnosine to my diabetic patients. Carnosine is found at most health food stores.

Benfotiamine

Benfotiamine is a fat-soluble form of vitamin B_1 and has been shown to help prevent the development as well as progression of many diabetic complications. This has been used in Europe for decades as a prescription medication. It helps to slow the progression of diabetic nerve, kidney, and retinal disease and also helps to relieve diabetic neuropathy. Benfotiamine is fat soluble, so it can easily enter cells and help prevent dysfunction associated with diabetes within the cells.

A recent double-blind study in Germany found that diabetic patients with polyneuropathy who were given 100 milligrams of benfotiamine four times a day for three weeks had statistically significant improvement in nerve function scores.[15]

Benfotiamine offers protection for the nerves, kidneys, retina, and vascular system from damage caused by diabetes. That is why supplementation is extremely important in preventing long-term complications of type 1 and type 2 diabetes. My recommended dose is 100 milligrams four times a day.

A Final Note

As you have observed, there are many nutrients and supplements that can help you effectively battle diabetes. If you are a type 2 diabetic and choose to follow this program and monitor your blood sugar, you should find that it is likely to drop within the normal range in a few months.

If you are a type 1 diabetic, research in islet cell transplants looks promising, or until you receive complete divine healing from God, you will always be on insulin. However, you may be able to lower your dosage of insulin by following the measures I have outlined. Regularly consult with

DR. COLBERT'S DIABETIC PROTOCOL

In addition to the protocol outlined in this chapter, I typically add supplements to prevent glycation, an extremely important aspect of preventing the long-term complications of diabetes. I generally add supplements such as carnosine, pyridoxal 5-phosphate, or benfotiamine. I usually start pyridoxal 5-phosphate (pyridoxamine, which used to be available, is no longer available here in the United States) if they are developing symptoms of glycation, such as kidney disease, neuropathy, or retinopathy. For more information on supplements, please refer to my book *The New Bible Cure for Diabetes*.

your physician; use these vitamins and nutrients as he or she may recommend. God has created these wonderful natural substances to empower us to maintain good health and to prevent or overcome the debilitating complications of diabetes.

Chapter 21

SUPPLEMENTS THAT SUPPORT
WEIGHT LOSS

Ever watch *The Red Green Show*? The off-beat series features Steve Smith as Red Green, who interacts with his hapless nephew, Harold, and a cast of wacky characters at Possum Lodge. Even though they stopped filming new episodes in 2006, reruns still air on Canadian television, the Comedy Network, and various Public Broadcasting System channels. Red is always looking for shortcuts to car repairs, home improvements, or unusual inventions, usually winding up with fractured, rib-tickling results. His solution to every problem: duct tape. He calls it the handyman's secret weapon.

Too many people are equally naive when it comes to fixing their weight and diabetes problems. Instead of duct tape, they think either a certain diet pill will do the trick or that downing the latest health drink a few times a day will suddenly make the pounds disappear. Many people are looking in vain for a magic pill that will enable them to eat anything they want, never exercise, and still lose weight. To quote an old cliché: "It ain't gonna happen."

Sure, things like amphetamines may appear to do the trick for a while. They suppress appetite and accelerate metabolism, allowing you to temporarily lose weight. However, the adverse reactions can be extreme: insomnia, nervousness, palpitations, headaches, arrhythmias, angina, heart attack, stroke, hypertension, hostility, aggressive behavior, and addiction, to name a few. Amphetamines may also worsen depression and anxiety. When you stop taking them, the reactions can be as severe as those I just listed. One common withdrawal response among users: regaining the weight they lost—and more.

Searching for the Magic Bullet

For years doctors, researchers, pharmaceutical companies, and nutritional companies have hunted for "The Pill to End All Diets." In the early 1990s researchers believed they had found it through combining two appetite suppressants—phentermine and fenfluramine. Known as fen-phen, this combo effectively suppressed appetite and became a hit. Individuals lost weight and kept it off as long as they continued on the medication. Studies revealed stunning results: on average, most users lost almost 16 percent of their body weight in just eight months. As an example, that correlates to a 200-pound person losing an impressive 32 pounds.

As you would expect, these results stimulated the formation of weight-loss clinics across America, where doctors prescribed this miracle pill combo. Yet after only a few years of use, a small percentage of users died of an extremely rare disease called primary pulmonary hypertension (PPH). This affected several patients out of one hundred thousand; about half of them

WILLING TO PAY

Sales of weight-loss drugs in the United States have surpassed the $1 billion mark, crossing that threshold in the fall of 2010.[1]

eventually required a heart-lung transplant to survive. To their credit, drug companies immediately pulled the two fenfluramine drugs, Pondimin and its derivative, Redux, off the market. However, authorities found phentermine to be relatively safe.

A few years later supplement companies once again believed they had found the magic pill, combining the herb ephedra with caffeine. This also proved to be a powerful formula for turning down the appetite and burning fat. Again, over the years both the effectiveness and the safety of ephedra were called into question. Ephedra has been linked to severe side effects, including arrhythmias, heart attack, stroke, hypertension, psychosis, seizure, and even death. To show what a major concern this is, consider a single statistic from the National Institutes of Health: products containing ephedra comprise less than 1 percent of all dietary supplement sales. Yet those products are responsible for an incredible 64 percent of adverse reactions from dietary supplements.[2]

Due to safety concerns, in 2004 the Food and Drug Administration (FDA) banned ephedra products in the United States. Although a federal court later upheld the ban, companies wiggle around it by selling extracts that contain little or no ephedrine. And some related herbs, such as bitter orange (citrus aurantium) and country mallow, remain on the market. Like ephedra, bitter orange supplements have been linked to stroke, cardiac arrest, angina, heart attack, ventricular arrhythmias, and death. These products are potentially lethal. I do not recommend them unless taken under the direction and close monitoring of a knowledgeable physician.

Among other herbs of concern is aristolochia, which is found in some Chinese herbal weight-loss supplements and may not even be listed as an ingredient. Aristolochia is a known kidney toxin and carcinogen in humans. There are also products containing usnea (usnic acid), a lichen for weight loss that can cause severe liver toxicity. In addition, some Brazilian diet pills have been found to be contaminated with amphetamines and other prescription drugs.[3]

Meant to Supplement, Not Replace

I hope by now you understand that for every supposed magic weight-loss pill, potential dangerous side effects loom close by. Unfortunately these often remain undiscovered until thousands—if not millions—of hopeful dieters have taken them. A few users have died. Let me remind you, the foundation for weight loss is simple: a healthy dietary plan and regular physical activity. The primary reason people are overweight or obese is too much calorie intake and too little physical activity. Period.

A weight-loss supplement is a nutritional product or herb intended to assist your healthy eating and activity plan with the ultimate goal of losing weight. A supplement comes alongside; it does not replace. Do not be deceived by crafty marketing that promises otherwise. Weight-loss and dietary supplements are not subject to the same standards as prescription drugs or medications sold over the counter. They can be marketed with only limited proof of safety or effectiveness.

ALLI AND HYDROXYCUT SIDE EFFECTS

Alli, one of the most common over-the-counter diet pills, may cause bowel changes in its users. These changes, which result from undigested fat going through the digestive system, may include gas with an oily discharge, loose stools or diarrhea, more frequent and urgent bowel movements, and hard-to-control bowel movements.

Hydroxycut products were recalled in May 2009 after reports of deadly liver failure and disease in individuals who took the products to lose weight. According to the *World Journal of Gastroenterology*, an ingredient in Hydroxycut from a fruit called *Garcinia cambogia* caused the liver disease and failure.[4]

However, there are a number of safe and fairly effective dietary supplements that look promising for weight loss. Each supplement has its own unique mechanism of action for weight loss, with some having more than one. I have categorized these beneficial and proven supplements into the following categories:

- Thermogenic agents (fat-burning agents)
- Appetite suppressants

- Supplements to increase satiety
- Supplements to improve insulin sensitivity
- Supplements to increase energy production

There are many causes of obesity; however, aging is one of the most common. This is because of a decrease in energy expenditure associated with aging. According to scientists, this may cause the body to store 120 to 190 excess calories daily. This may mean an extra 13 to 20 pounds of extra body fat a year.[5] Since there are many causes of obesity, I recommend adding a few safe nutritional supplements that work through different mechanisms, such as thermogenic agents, natural appetite suppressants that increase satiety, supplements that increase insulin sensitivity, and energy products. In treating hypertension, heart disease, diabetes, and other diseases, doctors add different medications with different mechanisms of action because when they are combined, their action is synergetic and more powerful. We now have safe, natural supplements that work by different mechanisms in helping individuals lose weight. Combining these will usually increase their effectiveness.

GREEN IS GOOD

A study found that after three months of taking green tea extract, overall body weight declined 4.6 percent while waist circumference decreased by nearly 4.5 percent.[6]

Thermogenic (Fat-Burning) Agents

The term *thermogenic* describes the body's natural means of raising its temperature to burn off more calories. More specifically, thermogenesis is the process of triggering the body to burn white body fat, which is the kind of fat we often accumulate as we age—the kind we typically see in overweight or obese people. Thermogenic agents, then, are fat burners that help to increase the rate of white body fat breakdown. Fortunately, most unsafe thermogenic agents have been pulled off the market.

Green tea

Green tea and green tea extract are my favorite weight-loss supplements. Green tea has been used for thousands of years in Asia as both a tea and an herbal medicine. It has two key ingredients: a catechin called epigallocatechin gallate (EGCG) and caffeine. Both lead to the release of more epinephrine, which then increases the metabolic rate. Ultimately, green tea promotes fat oxidation, which is fat burning. It also increases the rate at which you burn calories over a twenty-four-hour period.

An effective daily dose of EGCG is 90 milligrams or more, which can be consumed by drinking three or four cups of green tea a day. Do not add sugar, honey, or artificial sweeteners to it, though you may use the natural sweetener stevia.

Italian researchers created a green tea phytosome by combining green tea polyphenols with phospholipids, which caused a significant increase in the absorption of the polyphenols, including EGCG. A clinical trial involved one hundred significantly overweight subjects. Half the group received the green tea phytosome in a dose of two 150-milligram tablets daily. Both groups were placed on a reduced-calorie diet (1,850 calories a day for men and 1,350 calories a day for women). However, after forty-five days, the control group lost an average of 4 pounds and the green tea phytosome group lost an average of 13 pounds, about triple the control group. After ninety days, the control group lost an average of 9.9 pounds; the green tea group lost 30.1 pounds. The green tea phytosome group saw a 10 percent decrease of waist circumference, but the control group only realized a 5 percent reduction.[7] In addition to drinking green tea, I recommend 100 milligrams of green tea phytosome three times a day. (See Appendix B.)

Fucoxanthin

Derived from various types of edible seaweed, this carotenoid was traditionally known for its antioxidant powers. However, research in recent years has uncovered another major benefit to fucoxanthin: weight loss. Although early studies done exclusively on animals caused many critics to discredit claims of effectiveness in burning human fat, more recent ones involving human subjects are shifting opinions. Evidence of one such study found that combining fucoxanthin and pomegranate seed oil significantly increases metabolism. After sixteen weeks, researchers reported that those using the combination supplement had lost 15 pounds, compared to an average of a 3-pound loss by those taking a placebo.[8]

As we age, our metabolic rate naturally decreases, which prompts more storage of white body fat. Most people automatically turn to diets to solve this problem. But what they often overlook is that aging brings a decline in our *resting* metabolic rate, meaning that the white body fat that we naturally store isn't burned as quickly while we are sedentary. For this reason fucoxanthin appears to be a good supplement that can increase resting energy, decrease abdominal and liver fat storage, and ultimately reduce body weight.[9] A commonly recommended dose of fucoxanthin is 5 milligrams, taken three times a day. You can find this supplement in most health food stores.

Thyroid Support

All diabetics and obese patients should be screened for hypothyroidism, including the blood tests TSH, Free T3, Free T4, and thyroid peroxidase antibodies to rule out Hashimoto's thyroiditis, the most common cause of low thyroid. If a patient has low body temperature (less than 98 degrees), they most likely have a sluggish metabolism and may have sluggish thyroid function.

It's especially important to optimize the Free T3 blood level to improve the metabolic rate. The normal range of T3, according to the lab I use, is 2.1 to 4.4. I try to optimize the T3 level to a range of 3.0 to 4.2 by using Liothyronine or Armor Thyroid. I can sometimes optimize the T3 levels with natural supplements including Metabolic Advantage or iodine supplements. (See Appendix B.)

I also commonly perform a lab test to see if a patient is low in iodine before starting iodine supplements. According to the American Thyroid Association, 40 percent of the world's population is at risk for iodine deficiency.[10]

Appetite Suppressants

These supplements generally act on the central nervous system to decrease appetite or create a sensation of fullness. Although some medications in this category include risk-prone phenylpropanolamine (found in such products as Dexatrim), I have found a few safe, natural supplements that are extremely effective appetite suppressants.

WHAT'S THE POINT IF A PILL CAN DO IT?

Marketing researchers have found that the more proven a drug is to be effective at shedding pounds, the more lax the efforts of the user at continuing to eat well and exercise. Those who take prescription or over-the-counter diet pills are more likely to engage in eating junk food and living a sedentary lifestyle.[11]

L-tryptophan and 5-HTP

L-tryptophan and 5-hydroxy-tryptophan (commonly known as 5-HTP) are amino acids that help to manufacture serotonin. Serotonin assists in controlling carbohydrate and sugar cravings. L-tryptophan and 5-HTP also function like natural antidepressants. If you are taking migraine medications called triptans or SSRI (selective serotonin reuptake inhibitors) antidepressants, you should talk with your physician before taking either supplement. The typical dose of L-tryptophan is 500 to 2,000 milligrams at bedtime. For 5-HTP it is typically 50 to 100 milligrams one to three times a day or 100 to 300 milligrams at bedtime. Serotonin Max is an excellent supplement that helps boost serotonin levels naturally. (See Appendix B.)

L-tyrosine, N-acetyl L-tyrosine, and L-phenylalanine

L-tyrosine, N-acetyl L-tyrosine, and L-phenylalanine are naturally occurring amino acids found in numerous protein foods, including cottage cheese, turkey, and chicken. They help to raise norepinephrine and dopamine levels in the brain, which then helps decrease appetite and cravings and improves your mood. (SAM-e is another amino acid that helps raise norepinephrine and dopamine levels.) Doses of L-tyrosine, N-acetyl L-tyrosine, and L-phenylalanine may range from 500 to 2,000 milligrams a day (sometimes higher), but they should be taken on an empty stomach. I prefer N-acetyl L-tyrosine for most of my patients since the body absorbs it better than L-tyrosine or L-phenylalanine. I typically start patients on 500 to 1,000 milligrams of N-acetyl L-tyrosine, taken thirty minutes before breakfast and thirty minutes before lunch. I do not recommend taking any of these supplements in late afternoon because they may interfere with sleep. (See Appendix B.)

> **FIBER AWAY!**
>
> In addition to PGX, another great fiber for weight loss is glucomannan, made from the Asian root konjac. Glucomannan is five times more effective in lowering cholesterol when compared to other fibers such as psyllium, oat fiber, or guar gum. Because it expands to ten times its original size when placed in water, it is a great supplement to take before a meal to reduce your appetite as it expands in your stomach, but you should take it with 16 ounces of water or unsweetened black or green tea.

Supplements to Increase Satiety

Although I previously discussed fiber in chapter 11, it is worth a reminder that this valuable tool in the fight against diabetes helps control blood sugar and weight. Fiber supplements and foods high in fiber increase feelings of fullness by using several different mechanisms. Fiber slows the passage of food through the digestive tract, decreases the absorption of sugars and starches into the stomach, and expands and fills up the stomach—turning down the appetite. Although the American Heart Association and the National Cancer Institute recommend 30 grams or more of fiber each day, the average American only consumes between 12 and 17 grams.[12]

When it comes to losing weight and managing blood sugar levels, a little fiber goes a long way. One study found that consuming an extra 14 grams of soluble fiber each day for only two days was associated with a 10 percent decrease in caloric intake.[13] Soluble fiber supplements significantly increase post-meal satisfaction and should be taken before each meal to assist in weight loss. Soluble fiber lowers the blood sugar, slowing down digestion and the absorption of sugars and carbohydrates. This allows for a more gradual rise in blood sugar, which lowers the glycemic index of the foods you eat. This helps to improve the blood sugar levels.

The fiber that I prefer for weight-loss patients is PGX. I start with one capsule, taken with 8 to 16 ounces of water before each meal and snack, and then gradually increase the dose to two to four capsules until patients can control their appetite. Always take PGX with evening meals and snacks. (See Appendix B.)

Supplement to Increase Energy Production

L-carnitine is an amino acid that functions as a transporter of energy by shuttling fatty acids into the mitochondria, which act as our cells' energy factories by burning fatty acids for energy. In essence, L-carnitine helps our bodies turn food into energy. Humans synthesize very little carnitine, so we may need to supplement from outside sources. This applies especially to obese and older individuals, who typically have lower levels of carnitine than the average-weight segment of the population. As you might expect, individuals with insufficient carnitine have a greater difficulty burning fat for energy.

PGX FIBER

PGX, short for PolyGlycoPlex, is a unique blend of highly viscous fibers that act synergistically to create a much higher level of viscosity than the individual fibers alone. The viscosity is the gelling property. PGX absorbs hundreds of times its weight in water over one to two hours and expands in the digestive tract, creating a thick gelatinous material. It creates a feeling of fullness, stabilizes the blood sugar and insulin levels, and stabilizes appetite hormones.

PGX lowers blood sugar after eating by about 20 percent and lowers insulin secretion by about 40 percent. Researchers have found that higher doses of PGX can decrease appetite significantly. PGX works similar to gastric banding and has fewer gastrointestinal side effects than other viscous dietary fibers. However, start slowly or you may develop gas.

Taking soluble fiber before meals helps you feel satisfied sooner and usually decreases the amount of calories you consume. One study showed that 7 grams of the supplement psyllium before a meal decreased hunger and food intake while stabilizing blood sugar and insulin levels. In fact, special fiber blends, such as glucomannan, xanthan, and alginate (PGX), appear to be more effective than taking a single type of soluble fiber. In another study, participants took six PGX capsules before every meal. By the end of the three-week study, those taking the PGX had decreased their body fat by 2.8 percent.[14]

Milk, meat, fish, and cheese are good sources of L-carnitine, while mutton and lamb are also rich in this amino acid. In supplement form, I recommend combining L-carnitine with lipoic acid, PQQ (pyrroloquinoline quinone), and a glutathione-boosting supplement to increase energy production. A glutathione-boosting supplement will help quench free radicals in the mitochondria, including hydroxyl and hydrogen peroxide, which in turn helps to increase ATP production and one's energy. PQQ is a powerful antioxidant that protects the mitochondria from oxidative damage and actually stimulates the growth of new mitochondria. The mitochondria are, figuratively speaking, the energy factories in our cells that produce ATP which is our energy currency. Some cells such as the myocardial cells (heart muscle cells) have thousands of mitochondria, and other cells such as fat cells only have a very few mitochondria. L-carnitine, acetyl-L-carnitine, lipoic acid, PQQ, as well as glutathione-boosting supplements are all important to protect the mitochondria, grow new mitochondria, quench oxidative damage to the mitochondria, and increase energy production. One form of carnitine, acetyl-L-carnitine, is also able to cross the blood brain barrier and increase the energy of brain cells. This has numerous neuroprotective benefits and helps to increase neurotransmitters in the brain. It also protects brain cells from the effects of stress.

Overall, I recommend taking a combination of L-carnitine and acetyl-L-carnitine, lipoic acid, PQQ, and a glutathione-boosting supplement. By increasing your energy, you will be more likely to exercise regularly and burn more fat. The best time to take these supplements is in the morning and early afternoon (before 3:00 p.m.) on an empty stomach. If you take them any later, these supplements can impair your sleep. (See Appendix B.)

Also, green tea supplements and N-acetyl L-tyrosine help to increase your energy.

Other Common Supplements to Assist With Weight Loss

Irvingia

Irvingia is a fruit-bearing plant grown in the jungles of Cameroon in Africa. Irvingia gabonensis helps to resensitize your cells to insulin. It appears to be able to reverse leptin resistance by lowering levels of C-reactive protein (CRP), an inflammatory mediator. In a double-blind study, 102 overweight participants received 150 milligrams of Irvingia or a placebo twice a day for ten weeks. At the end of the period, the Irvingia group lost an average of 28 pounds and the placebo group just 1 pound. The Irvingia group also lost an average 6.7 inches from their waistline and decreased total body fat by

18.4 percent. They also had a 26 percent reduction of total cholesterol, a 27 percent decrease in LDL (bad cholesterol), a 32 percent decrease in fasting blood sugar, and a 52 percent decrease in CRP.[15]

It is believed that Irvingia has the ability to enable one to lose weight by simply lowering CRP levels, which in turn lowers leptin resistance. Leptin is a hormone that tells your brain you've eaten enough and that it is time to stop. It also enhances your body's ability to use fat as an energy source. One also needs zinc, 12 to 15 milligrams a day, which is present in most comprehensive multivitamins, in order for leptin to function optimally.

Unfortunately, because of Americans' sedentary lifestyles and highly processed, high-glycemic food choices, many overweight and obese patients have acquired resistance to leptin. As a result, this hormone no longer works properly in their bodies. Similar to insulin resistance, leptin resistance is a chronic inflammatory condition that contributes to weight gain and belly fat. It is also critically important to follow the dietary program that I have outlined in this book, which is also an anti-inflammatory diet. Simply decreasing inflammatory foods enables most to start losing belly fat and also allows leptin to function optimally.

I have been using Irvingia with diabetic patients since 2008 and have seen remarkable improvements in most of their blood sugar measurements and hemoglobin A1c levels. The generally recommended dose is 150 milligrams of standardized Irvingia extract, twice a day.

Calcium

Both children and adults with a low calcium intake are more likely to gain weight or be overweight or obese when compared to individuals with a higher calcium intake. Dairy products, such as plain low-fat yogurt and kefir, that provide total calcium of 800 to 1,200 milligrams a day will help lower body fat, increase muscle mass, and ultimately help with weight loss. However, it's interesting to note that taking calcium supplements alone does not appear to help with weight loss.

The hoodia controversy

Hoodia is a South African plant similar to a cactus that may help suppress the appetite. Initially used by tribal leaders to enable them to go on long journeys without getting hungry, various sources cite thousands of years' worth of Bushman history to verify its effectiveness. Although these tribal hunters obviously have not conducted scientific studies to prove hoodia is an effective appetite suppressant, one 2001 clinical study by a company called Phytopharm found individuals who consumed the plant ate 1,000 fewer calories a day than those who didn't take hoodia.[16] One of the company's researchers, Richard Dixey, MD, explained that hoodia contains a molecule that is ten thousand times more active than glucose.[17]

However, there is a catch. When news of this supposed miracle supplement hit the headlines, dozens (if not hundreds) of companies started marketing hoodia—without having any actual hoodia in their products. The result was that more hoodia was "produced" in a single year than in all of African history—highly unlikely, to say the least. Even today, it is possible that much of what is sold in the United States either contains ineffective hoodia variations or no hoodia. So be wary of falling for marketing schemes with this substance.

In Summary

While some questionable products are on the market, there are a variety of safe, effective over-the-counter dietary supplements for weight loss. Some people may find that incorporating a combination of these into their eating and activity plan works even better. Others may not need to take any supplements. Most of my overweight and obese patients have found that drinking green tea or taking green tea phytosome, certain amino acids (such as Serotonin Max and N-acetyl L-tyrosine), and PGX fiber supplements before each meal and snack (especially in the evening) helped them shed pounds.

If you continue experiencing problems controlling your appetite or struggle with food cravings, decreased energy, or insulin resistance, you will likely require one or more of the supplements I just reviewed. The same goes if you do not feel full or satisfied after a meal or if you have low hormone levels. However, I remind you what I said earlier: supplements are just supplements, not magic pills. Excess weight was years in the making, so it won't suddenly vanish. The good news is you no longer have to be duped by wonder-working, flab-busting, "as seen on TV" promises. Armed with the right eating and activity plan, you can shed the weight and reverse diabetes.

Chapter 22

THE IMPORTANCE OF ACTIVITY

E*xercise*. Does that word fill you with dread and visions of boredom, fatigue, and your tongue hanging out as you gasp for air? If you hate working out, you are not alone. Even big-name celebrities who are known for their ultra-fit bodies and sex appeal disdain it. Singer and actress Janet Jackson says, "I hate working out—and hate is a strong word, but I cannot stand working out."[1] Bruce Willis, known for his tough-guy roles in numerous action-adventure flicks, admits, "I'm lazy, I hate working out, I only do it for films and I think of it as work."[2]

Nor is Willis the only Hollywood star with an aversion to exercise. Actress Katherine Heigl, best known for her Emmy Award–winning performances on *Grey's Anatomy*, says, "If I wasn't in this industry, I wouldn't work out. But I have hips and a butt and everything that goes along with that, including cellulite."[3]

From the world of athletics, listen to tennis star Serena Williams: "I hate working out more than anything, but I have to—when I'm running, I think about how much I want to win. That's the only thing that keeps me going....I guess everyone has to find that one thing that encourages them and just think about it the entire time you're working out. But I have to be honest, I hate going to the gym. I don't like running. I hate doing anything that has to do with working out."[4]

The one person you might have expected to champion exercise was fitness buff Jack LaLanne, who died in January of 2011 at age ninety-six. Even the legendary workout master once said, "I hate exercise, but I love the results."[5] Such quips illustrate our love-hate relationship with exercise. In particular, we dread taking the time out of our already cramped schedules for it. What other explanation is there for all the late-night TV infomercials about time-saving exercise gadgets promising pounds will "instantly" fall off if we use their product? We always want the quick solution.

As a result, two-thirds of all Americans are not physically active on a regular basis. Less than half get less than the recommended amount of exercise. Sadly, a full 25 percent—a quarter of the population!—get absolutely no exercise.[6] The leading reason, according to almost every survey conducted, places time at the top of its list of excuses.[7] People rationalize they are just too busy to exercise. According to the CDC, the average adult, age eighteen to sixty-four, needs 150 minutes (2.5 hours) a week of moderate aerobic activity and two or more days a week of muscle-strengthening activity.[8] A recent study found that women over forty-five years of age need 60 minutes of moderate exercise a day to prevent weight gain as they aged, even with consuming a normal diet.[9]

What's in a Word?

While you may not think you have the time, exercise is essential for good health. That applies to every human being—especially anyone hoping to shed weight and reverse diabetes. You can restrict your diet and eat less than your daily requirement. Yet without burning off calories through physical activity, you have only completed half the weight-loss equation. After working with thousands of overweight, obese, and type 2 diabetic individuals, I have discovered that almost without exception, they struggle with a perception of exercise. And, it all comes down to that single word: *exercise*.

> **MARATHON BURN**
>
> To burn off the 1,510 calories in a Quiznos large Chicken Carbonara, you'd have to expend the same calories it takes to bike across the state of Delaware (thirty miles).[10]

For many, *exercise* conjures up the same negative feelings as *diet*. Those who are overweight or obese think of exercise in terms of pain, sweating, humiliation, embarrassment, and anxiety. They may visualize themselves in a health club surrounded by people with perfect bodies, a physical education instructor testing their lack of physical capabilities, or an overbearing coach from their youth. Because this word often stimulates dread, I use a different one: *activity*. To some, this seems a bit silly. It's just a word, after all—what difference could substituting one word make? Isn't it still referring to the same thing?

I cannot explain why this works, but it does. *Activity* seems less intrusive; it doesn't trigger emotional symptoms or anxiety. For most overweight or obese individuals, it is safe and nonthreatening. It does not overwhelm them with thoughts of time commitments, discipline, or early-morning alarm clocks.

It is up to you whether you adapt a change of vocabulary. However, the bigger issue you cannot overlook is that both a change of diet and regular activity are crucial for weight loss. Plain and simple, the reason why people successfully lose weight and keep it off is because they are physically active.

The Perks of Regular Activity

In case you needed a reminder, here are some of many benefits that come with regular activity:

- It decreases the risk of heart disease, stroke, and the development of hypertension.
- It helps prevent type 2 diabetes.
- It helps protect you from developing certain types of cancer.
- It helps prevent osteoporosis and aids in maintaining healthy bones.
- It helps prevent arthritis and aids in maintaining healthy joints.
- It slows down the overall aging process.
- It improves your mood and reduces the symptoms of anxiety and depression.
- It increases energy and mental alertness.
- It improves digestion.
- It gives you more restful sleep.
- It helps prevent colds and flu.
- It alleviates pain.
- And the favorite reason among overweight and obese people... it promotes weight loss and decreases appetite.

However, there's more. Exercise holds special benefits for diabetics. Multiple studies have shown that those who have a physically active lifestyle are less prone to develop type 2 diabetes. I believe this is because physical exercise battles the root of type 2 diabetes, which is insulin resistance or when muscle cells lose their sensitivity to insulin. Research has shown that your muscle cells are much less likely to become resistant to insulin if you keep them fit through regular exercise.

Studies have also shown that regular exercise improves glucose tolerance and lowers blood sugar as well as insulin requirements. The more muscle tissue we develop in our large muscle groups such as the thighs and buttocks, the more sugar we remove from the bloodstream. Generally speaking, the greater the muscle mass, especially in the large muscle groups, the larger the corresponding drop in insulin resistance. Also, by burning calories, exercise helps control weight, an important factor in the management of type 2 diabetes.

A study at the Cooper Institute for Aerobics Research in Dallas shows that staying fit may be the most important thing you can do to avoid type 2 diabetes. The researchers put 8,633 men, average age forty-three, through a treadmill test. Then, six years later, they screened them for diabetes. The men who scored poorly on the fitness test were almost four times more likely to have developed the disease than those who did well on the treadmill. These scores turned out to be the most accurate predictor of diabetes—more than age, obesity, high blood pressure, or family history.[11]

Don't use Hollywood stars or fitness gurus as an excuse to justify a lack of activity. When push comes to shove, you must do your part and get moving regularly. This takes courage. If it didn't, everyone would do it. You must take the offensive to battle and hopefully reverse diabetes, remembering that it is a scourge that can weaken and damage other organs in your body.

The Natural Weight-Loss Supplement

There is no better way to complement a weight-loss dietary and supplement program than physical activity. How does it help? The ways are as plentiful as the many benefits I just listed. First, it helps raise the metabolic rate during and after the activity. It enables you to develop more muscle, which raises the metabolic rate all day—even while you sleep. It decreases body fat and improves your ability to cope with stress by lowering the stress hormone cortisol.

Such activity also raises serotonin levels, which helps reduce cravings for sweets and carbohydrates. It assists in burning off dangerous belly fat and improves your body's ability to handle sugar. Finally, regular physical activity can even help control your appetite by boosting serotonin levels, lowering cortisol, and decreasing insulin levels (which can also decrease your chances for insulin resistance).

> **STRENGTH IN YEARS**
>
> In 2004 Connecticut resident George Brunstad became the oldest man to swim the English Channel when he crossed the twenty-five-mile stretch at age seventy. Though he swam an extra seven miles due to strong currents, Brunstad completed the grueling journey just a minute shy of sixteen hours. Just as admirable was the former pilot's underlying purpose for swimming, which was to let people know about a ministry his church sponsors in Haiti.[12]

There are numerous enjoyable activities to choose from; for example, cycling, swimming, working out on an elliptical machine, dancing, and hiking. Sports such as basketball, volleyball, soccer, football, racquetball, tennis, and squash are all considered aerobic. Pilates, ballroom dancing, washing the car by hand, working in your yard, and mowing the grass qualify too—anything that raises the heart rate enough to burn fat.

A great aerobic activity is brisk walking, although for diabetic patients with foot ulcers or numbness in the feet, walking is not the best activity. In its place they should try cycling, an elliptical machine, or pool activities while inspecting the feet before and after activity. If you can walk, to enter your target heart rate zone, walk briskly enough so that you cannot sing and slowly enough so that you can talk. Following this formula is one reason that I recommend people find an activity partner to talk with them as they walk. (Skeptics might say that misery loves company.)

Here are a few other tips to get you started:

- Choose something that is fun and enjoyable. You will never stick to any activity program if you dread or hate it.

- Wear comfortable, well-fitting shoes and socks.

- If you are a type 1 diabetic, you will need to work with your doctor in order to adjust insulin doses while increasing your activity. Realize that exercising will lower your blood sugar; this can be potentially dangerous in a type 1 diabetic.

Muscles, Metabolism, and Aging

Everyone wants to look young and fit forever. That's particularly true in the United States, where we plaster buff, sculpted, trimmed, toned, and youthful bodies all over magazine covers, TV ads, and movie screens. Great looks hide the reality that adults typically lose ½ to 1 pound of muscle tissue every year after the age of twenty-five, meaning our bodies naturally progress toward more fat and less muscle. That isn't the greatest news for those overloaded with fat. However, such a realization can be a driving force to shape up. The more muscle mass, generally the higher your metabolic rate and the more calories you will burn at rest. For each pound of muscle mass that you either gain or do not lose, you will burn between 30 and 50 calories a day.

I will never forget the patient I saw years ago during residency. The star running back on a high school football team, he had fractured his left thigh. Part of the reason he played running back was the power in his legs. Not surprisingly, his thighs were extremely muscular. Before, he said, he had been able to leg press more than 1,000 pounds for ten repetitions. Because of his injury, though, this athlete had to wear a full leg cast for approximately two months.

When we removed the cast, we were shocked at how much his left leg had atrophied. Measuring his thighs showed a 32-inch circumference around his mid-right thigh; his left checked in at a mere 24 inches. In only two months, inactivity had cost this young man 8 inches of muscle. A similar process occurs with most adults, though not as quickly. Yet if you are inactive, your muscles are slowly melting away. Your metabolic rate is decreasing, and muscle tissue is (typically) being replaced with fat. Many people do not notice because the size of their arm or leg remains the same, when in fact it is simply a case of fat replacing muscle tissue—similar to the marbling of meat.

This is particularly true for women. A woman's metabolism typically begins to decrease at age twenty at a rate of about 5 percent per decade. To understand this, let's use the example of an average fifty-year-old female— I'll call her Sarah. Since her late twenties, Sarah's weight has slowly increased from around 120 pounds to her current weight of 150. During those years she gained 30 pounds of fat while losing 15 to 30 pounds of muscle. That may sound like it averages out, except when you consider the corresponding drop in metabolic rate.

At twenty, Sarah could eat 2,000 calories a day and maintain her 120-pound frame. At the age of fifty, if she eats 2,000 calories a day, she will most likely gain weight because of this lost muscle tissue. Why? For each pound of muscle tissue lost, your metabolic rate decreases 30 to 50 calories per day. So in addition to losing 15 pounds of muscle, Sarah lost the ability to burn 450 to 750 more calories a day.

Can you see why maintaining or gaining muscle mass is so crucial? Muscle does not just look better than fat; it is essential for maintaining a healthy body. The only way to keep muscle intact is to use it and strengthen it, which means increasing your activity level. When you remain inactive, you put yourself in a body cast—so to speak—as your metabolic rate nosedives and you slowly morph into a fat magnet.

Recommended Amount of Activity

Once I have persuaded patients they need more activity, their next question is: How much do I need? Unfortunately, no universal number applies. There are numerous factors involved in engaging in activity to lose weight, starting with the heart.

Every activity either requires or can be performed at different levels of intensity. Given that, it makes sense that every person hoping to lose weight has an ideal intensity at which he or she should work out. This is called your target heart rate zone, which generally ranges from 65 to 85 percent of your maximum heart rate.

To calculate the low end of this zone, start by subtracting your age from

220. This is your maximum heart rate. For example, for someone forty years old the formula is:

220 – 40 = 180 beats per minute

Multiply this number by 65 percent to find the low end of the target heart rate zone:

180 x 0.65 = 117 beats per minute

To figure out the high end of the zone, multiply maximum heart rate by 85 percent, or:

180 x 0.85 = 153 beats per minute

So, if you are forty, you should keep your heart rate between 117 and 153 beats per minute when exercising. However, that is quite a wide range, which prompts the next question: Which end of the zone do you aim for to lose weight? Experts have debated this ever since the "target zone" idea came into being many years ago. To find the answer, let's look at the types of activity that push the heart to these two extremes.

Burning Fat With Aerobic Activity

The word *aerobic* means "in the presence of air or oxygen." Aerobic activity is simply movement that strengthens the lungs and the heart. It involves steady, continuous movements that work large muscle groups in repetitive motion for at least twenty minutes. The key point for weight loss with aerobic activity is to maintain a moderate pace, which triggers your body to burn fat as its preferred fuel.

One of the most common workout mistakes I see among overweight people is their tendency to jump on a treadmill and run as hard as they can for as long as possible. They intend to burn off more fat by doing this, but in the long run (pardon my pun), they won't. Sprinting, running, or jogging at high intensity for so long you are short of breath actually makes you burn less fat as fuel. For inactive individuals who are just starting to work out, it's also the quickest way to burnout.

NOT JUST NERVOUS

Fidgeting or getting up from your seat frequently can cause you to burn an additional 350 calories a day—which amounts to 36 pounds lost in a year![13]

Remember, aerobic means with oxygen; therefore, the activity you choose must be of moderate intensity for your body to use oxygen in order to burn the fat as fuel. When you exercise to the point that you are severely short of breath, you are no longer performing aerobically. Instead you have shifted to an anaerobic activity, which means activity without oxygen. Anaerobic activity burns glycogen—stored sugar—as primary fuel instead of fat. When you run out of glycogen and have not eaten for a while, you may begin breaking down muscle tissue and burning muscle protein as fuel. (Notice that I haven't yet mentioned burning fat.) Many marathoners and triathletes burn a significant amount of muscle as fuel, which is often why they remain so lean.

If you are overweight and aim to burn primarily fat, you need to work out at a moderate intensity of 65 to 85 percent of your maximum heart rate. This is the fat-burning range of your target heart rate zone. As you approach the high end, you near anaerobic activity, which does less good in burning fat. This might be a completely revolutionary idea. If so, it may be a struggle to change. Most people believe that to the hardest worker—meaning the guy who runs the fastest and sweats the most—go the spoils. Not true. If you are overweight or obese, working out at a higher intensity for long stretches may not only sabotage your fat-burning ability, it may also increase cortisol levels, which can cause more belly fat to accumulate.

INTERVAL TRAINING

High-intensity interval training (HIIT) mixes high-intensity bursts of exercise with moderate-intensity recovery periods, usually for a period of less than twenty minutes. It is used mostly for individuals trying to lose weight.

When starting any activity program, work out around 65 percent of your maximum heart rate. As you become more aerobically conditioned, gradually increase the intensity to 70 percent of maximum heart rate. After a few more weeks, increase to 75 percent, and so on. You may never be able to work out at 85 percent of maximum rate, especially if you are huffing and puffing. Be sure that as you increase the intensity of your workouts, you remain able to converse with another person. That is a fairly good sign that you are training aerobically and are burning fat. When you are in good aerobic condition, you can start interval training.

High-Intensity Interval Training

Researchers at McMaster University have found that brief sessions of high-intensity workouts were able to lower blood sugar levels rapidly in type 2 diabetics. This is the first study to show that intense interval training may be a powerful, time-efficient strategy to improve blood sugar regulation in individuals with type 2 diabetes. Each workout consisted of riding a stationary bike for ten bouts of sixty seconds at about 90 percent of the maximum heart rate, with one minute of casual riding between each burst of exercise. The workout also included a warm-up and a cool-down so that each training session had only twenty-five minutes of total exercise time. The participants did three twenty-five-minute workouts a week. These workouts lowered twenty-four-hour blood sugar concentrations, decreased blood sugar spikes after meals, and increased skeletal muscle mitochondrial capacity, a marker of metabolic health.[14]

If you have type 2 diabetes and have exercised for a month or longer or achieved good aerobic conditioning, you should consider high-intensitiy interval training. Just three sessions of twenty-five minutes a week is all you need. Be sure to have a physical exam with your physician, including an EKG, before starting a high-intensity interval training program. Also consider having a stress test.

How Much?

This brings us back to the original question: How much activity? A 2004 Duke University study shed some light on this. Over a period of eight months, researchers at Duke studied a group of overweight men and women ages forty to sixty-five. Participants were split into four main groups: those who walked twelve miles a week, those who jogged twelve miles a week, those who jogged twenty miles a week, and those who did nothing. None of the groups changed anything about their diets. All exercised at different maximum heart rates. As you might expect, the sedentary group gained weight, added to their waistlines, and upped their body fat percentage. Those who walked twelve miles a week (or thirty minutes a day) did so at 40 to 55 percent of their maximum heart rate. Their results were minimal. The group that jogged this same distance each day kept their heart rates between 65 and 80 percent the maximum rate, meaning they exercised within their target heart rate zone. Though some of their results were similar to the walking group, they did lose more body fat and gained more lean muscle. Finally, those who jogged for twenty miles each week kept within their target heart rate zone and saw by far the best results. On average, the

> **DOG LOVERS?**
>
> Approximately 60 percent of dog owners do not walk their dogs, simply letting them out in the backyard.[16]

members of this group dropped 3.5 percent of their weight, 3.4 percent of their waist measurement, 4.9 percent of body fat measurements, and added 1.4 percent of lean muscle.[15]

Clearly, it pays to be active. The longer you engage in activity at a moderate intensity, the more fat you burn as fuel. I am not suggesting you have to jog twenty miles a week. Still, you can start by choosing enjoyable, fun activities that you and your family can do daily to obtain similar results. Unless you have already been working out, I suggest that you initially set a goal of twenty minutes a day, which may be split into ten minutes, twice a day. (You can do this by simply walking your dog!) Once you have adapted, gradually increase to thirty minutes and eventually forty minutes or more. To minimize soreness, get activity every other day, three days a week, and work up to five or six days a week. And remember, a brisk walk can accomplish almost as much as jogging—provided you maintain 65 to 85 percent of your maximum heart rate.

Resistance Exercises

Resistance training usually involves lifting weights to build muscles. I have shared this simple rule of thumb with my diabetic patients for years: the more muscle you build in the lower extremities and buttocks, generally the better your blood sugar control.

Scientific studies have proven that a combination of resistance training and aerobic exercise is the most effective way to improve insulin sensitivities in diabetics.[17] That is why I call aerobic activity and resistance training a one-two punch to knock out type 2 diabetes. Aerobic activity combined with resistance training will improve blood sugar control even better than most diabetic medications, especially if high-intensity interval training is practiced regularly.

These strengthening activities include weight training with free weights or machines, calisthenics, Pilates, resistance band activities, core-specific activities, and balance ball activities. To eliminate the risk of injury, you must maintain good posture and form while performing these exercises. In addition, it is important to learn the correct lifting techniques, the correct range of motion, correct breathing, and the correct speed of the movement in which muscles are being trained.

THIGH CIRCUMFERENCE

Thin thighs (less than 24 inches in circumference) are associated with significantly increased risk of death and cardiovascular disease. The risk increases as thigh circumference decreases. This makes it important to maintain a thigh circumference greater than 24 inches.[18]

The thigh muscles are the largest in the body and need to be exercised both aerobically and with repetitive exercises. I have found that as my patients with diabetes increase the muscle mass in their thighs, their blood sugar typically decreases.

You should typically perform ten to twelve repetitions per set. When starting resistance training, I recommend only performing one set per activity. This reduces soreness, which is common in beginning any type of strengthening program. As you become better conditioned over time, you can increase to two or three sets per activity for each body part to strengthen and tone muscles. Remember, go slow! Strength training causes microscopic tears in muscle fibers, which eventually causes them to grow stronger and larger. This in turn increases your metabolic rate. Never overdo it, and train the same muscles every day; the muscles will not have time to repair and rebuild.

Eventually, after a couple of weeks of strength training, you will be able to increase your workouts to three or four days a week. By following the correct lifting techniques, you will prevent injury, build muscle, and burn fat. I recommend finding a certified personal trainer to teach you this valuable information so you can maximize results and prevent injury. After years of visiting health clubs, I am appalled at the large percentage of people who lift weights incorrectly.

Putting It All Together

To lose weight, you can literally start your activity program on the right foot. Unless you are physically restricted, walking is the easiest way to stay active. All you need for equipment are some comfortable clothes and a good pair of walking shoes. It's a great way to enjoy the outdoors. Follow my earlier recommendation to find an activity partner, and you can catch up on conversation while he or she holds you accountable with your exercise. Avoid the routine; for variety, go to a park or visit a hiking trail.

I believe in monitoring yourself. An excellent way to monitor the steps you walk during the day is by using a pedometer. I urge all my patients to get one and track their step count during the day. Typically a person walks 3,000 to 5,000 steps a day. To stay fit, set a goal of 10,000 steps, or approximately five miles. To lose weight, aim for between 12,000 and 15,000 steps per day. Other ways to reach this upper

KEEPING TRACK

Researchers say that self-monitoring devices, such as a pedometer, heart rate monitor, or even a simple exercise journal can account for a 25 percent increase in successfully controlling your weight.[19]

target: walking your dog, parking farther out in the parking lot at work or when shopping, and taking the stairs instead of the elevator whenever possible.

Before engaging in any activity, make sure that you have either eaten a meal two or three hours prior or have had a healthy snack about thirty to sixty minutes beforehand. It is never good to work out when hungry; you may end up burning muscle protein as energy—which is very expensive fuel. Losing muscle lowers your metabolic rate.

After you are into the routine of walking approximately thirty minutes, five or six days a week, or you are taking 12,000 steps a day on your pedometer, you can start resistance training. Before this routine, always do a five-minute warm-up by walking on a treadmill or elliptical machine or riding a stationary bike at low intensity. This increases blood flow to muscles and joints, prepares them for the workout, and significantly reduces the risk of injury.

Once you have warmed up, do a twenty- to thirty-minute workout, using free weights, machines, calisthenics, Pilates, or some other strengthening activity. This burns up much of the glycogen stored in the muscles and liver. Following this, you will be ready for a thirty-minute aerobic workout, such as brisk walking on a treadmill, cycling, or using an elliptical machine or other cardio equipment. This aerobic session allows you to mainly burn fat. Once you have become aerobically fit, consider starting high-intensity interval training.

When you are finished with both the strength and aerobic parts of your workout, cool down by doing a low-intensity aerobic activity for another five minutes—just like you warmed up. You may also want to do some stretching after your cool-down.

I recommend a resistance program three to four days a week, working out every other day for twenty to thirty minutes, and an aerobic program five to six days each week for at least thirty minutes. When you start high-intensity interval training, you only need three to four days a week for twenty-five to thirty minutes. Always warm up before any activity and cool down at the end. And keep things fun by periodically changing the routine. By varying your activities every month or so, you can shock your muscles into new growth—which means burning more fat. That is a step every diabetic should want to take.

FROM DON COLBERT

God desires to heal you of disease. His Word is full of promises that confirm His love for you and His desire to give you His abundant life. His desire includes more than physical health for you; He wants to make you whole in your mind and spirit as well as through a personal relationship with His Son, Jesus Christ.

If you haven't met my best friend, Jesus, I would like to take this opportunity to introduce Him to you. It is very simple. If you are ready to let Him come into your life and become your best friend, all you need to do is sincerely pray this prayer:

> *Lord Jesus, I want to know You as my Savior and Lord. I believe You are the Son of God and that You died for my sins. I also believe You were raised from the dead and now sit at the right hand of the Father praying for me. I ask You to forgive me for my sins and change my heart so that I can be Your child and live with You eternally. Thank You for Your peace. Help me to walk with You so that I can begin to know You as my best friend and my Lord. Amen.*

If you have prayed this prayer, you have just made the most important decision of your life. I rejoice with you in your decision and your new relationship with Jesus. Please contact my publisher at pray4me@charismamedia.com so that we can send you some materials that will help you become established in your relationship with the Lord. We look forward to hearing from you.

Appendix A

SIMPLE RULES

Ever attend a social gathering and steadily work your way through the buffet, collecting treats like a vacuum cleaner scoops up dust? You know the drill. It starts with several handfuls of potato, tortilla, or corn chips, stopping to enliven the taste with several spoonfuls of cheese, ranch, or French onion dip. Then it's on to the meat tray for a couple "small" sandwiches of roast beef or turkey, some tomato, a bit of Swiss and perhaps a little Colby, all topped off by a dollop of mayonnaise and a squirt of mustard. Oh, those stuffed mushrooms look good. So do the crab puffs. Those cherry tarts look delicious. And the miniature pecan pies…yummy!

Once you've worked your way through the line, chatted with several friends, and rested awhile, it's back for another sampling. Maybe some potato and macaroni salad, another few handfuls of chips, and some other tasty delight you missed the first time. After all, there's so much—you want to try a little bit of everything. All these salt-laden foods call for a thirst quencher too, whether it's a couple 20-ounce soft drinks or a sugary-sweet bottle of Snapple. Before you know it, your belly is protesting about the 2,000 or 3,000 calories worth of food you just crammed into it, even as you're thinking, "Why am I so stuffed? I just had a few snacks."

After reviewing the previous chapters about meal planning and snacks, I hope you have developed a more intentional mind-set toward daily food intake. Fail to take this step, and I guarantee you will fall prey to the office social gathering, family get-together, friend's birthday party, or one of the other calorie-, fat-, and salt-laden temptation-filled occasions that will regularly enter your life. Although I have already covered some of the following, in this chapter I want to review some of the recommendations I make to patients who need to lose weight, especially belly fat. I will go into more specifics later on, but to start, here are a dozen basic rules for quick reference. You may want to make a condensed copy of them to post on your desk or carry in your wallet or purse.

- Graze throughout the day (on salads and veggies, not chips and fatty treats).

- As I like to say, eat breakfast like a king, lunch like a prince, and dinner like a pauper.

- Eat smaller midmorning and midafternoon snacks, such as protein bars and coconut milk kefir blended with plant or whey protein.

- Avoid all simple-sugar foods, i.e., candies, cookies, cakes, pies, and doughnuts. If you must have sugar, use either stevia, xylitol, Sweet Balance, or Just Like Sugar (found in health food stores).

- Drink 1 to 2 quarts of filtered or bottled water a day. That includes 16 ounces thirty minutes before each meal, or one to two 8-ounce glasses two and a half hours after each meal. Also, drink 8 to 16 ounces of water upon awakening.

- Avoid alcohol.

- Avoid all fried foods.

- Avoid starches or at least decrease them dramatically. This includes all breads, crackers, bagels, potatoes, pasta, rice, and corn. Limit beans, peas, lentils, and sweet potatoes to a half cup, one to two times a day. Avoid bananas and dried fruit.

- Eat fresh, low-glycemic fruits only for breakfast or lunch and occasionally with morning and early afternoon snacks; eat steamed, stir-fried, or raw vegetables, lean meats, salads with colorful vegetables (preferably with a salad spritzer), almonds, and seeds.

- Take fiber supplements, such as two to three capsules of PGX fiber, with 8 to 16 ounces of water before each meal and two PGX fiber capsules with each snack.

- For snacks, choose bars such as Jay Robb bars, Nutiva Hemp Chocolate Bars, and Fitsmart bars. Try to limit these bars to one every day or every other day. These may be purchased at a health food store. (Refer to *Dr. Colbert's "I Can Do This" Diet* for more information.)

- Do not eat later than 7:00 p.m.

General Recommendations

Remember one of the most the important guidelines for weight loss that will help you reverse diabetes: eat every three to three and a half hours to keep your blood sugar levels stable, and remember to eat healthy, well-balanced snacks. Here are others:

- For meals, choose a lean protein, a low-glycemic carb, and a healthy fat (but make sure you go "carb free" and low fat after 6:00 p.m.).

- For morning snacks, the easiest thing to do is choose a piece of fruit from the Approved Foods chart in chapters 16 and 17. You may also choose from the afternoon snacks listed later in this chapter. As with meals, take two to three PGX fiber capsules with 16 ounces of water before or after your snack. It's best to drink green, white, or regular tea with your snacks, except for your evening snack. Remember to drink iced tea or water since that helps to boost the metabolic rate and will help you lose weight.

- For afternoon snacks, choose any of the approved snacks from Approved Foods or a "mini-meal" consisting of a half-serving of protein, a half-serving of low-glycemic carbs, and a half-serving of fat. Take one 5-HTP or Serotonin Max if craving sugar or carbs. And remember the PGX fiber capsules. (See Appendix B.)

- For evening snacks, choose any of the approved snacks listed later in this chapter or a "mini-meal" (leaving out the carbs and fats). You can find out more information on a "mini-meal" in my book *Dr. Colbert's "I Can Do This" Diet.*

- Serving sizes for protein are typically 2 to 6 ounces for women and 3 to 8 ounces for men.

- Limit red meat intake to a maximum of 18 ounces per week.

- All soups should be low sodium, vegetable or bean, and broth based, not cream based.

- Use Himalayan or Celtic sea salt instead of regular table salt (in small amounts, less than 1 teaspoon a day).

- It's best to avoid wheat and corn products. However, an occasional a slice of Ezekiel 4:9 bread toasted with breakfast or lunch every three to four days is acceptable.

- If desired, you may sweeten foods and beverages with stevia, xylitol, or Just Like Sugar. It is best to avoid artificial sweeteners such as NutraSweet and Splenda.

- You may add a small amount of organic skim milk to your coffee, if desired.

- If organic foods are too expensive, one option is to at least choose organic options for the meat or other protein you consume most often. If you aren't able to buy organic, then choose very lean cuts of meat, white chicken, or turkey meat; peel the skin off poultry; and thoroughly wash fruits and vegetables that cannot be peeled. Eat dairy rarely, similar to what you do with wheat and corn. Choose part-skim milk or low-fat cheese, nonfat cottage cheese or cream cheese, and plain or vanilla Greek yogurt. (Still, if you can tighten your budget to free up some room for organic or range-fed items, these are the best choices. For meats, Maverick Ranch or Applegate Farms are good choices. I recommend prepackaged nitrite-free turkey breast, chicken breast, ham, or lean roast beef slices.)

- I recommend large salads of colorful vegetables, tomatoes, raw carrots, onions, cucumbers, and other vegetables make up the majority of lunches and dinners. Save the salad for your evening meal if you are tired of eating salad at both meals.

- If you choose to make your smoothies with coconut milk, be sure that it only contains 80 calories per cup. (So Delicious is one brand that meets this criteria.) You may have to purchase it from a health food store; however, it is usually available at your local supermarket.

Recommended appliances (all are optional)

To save time on cooking and preparing meals, I recommend:

- George Foreman Next Grilleration Grill
- Vegetable steamer
- Blender

- Toaster
- Convection oven

Recommended nutritional supplements (all are optional)

You can experience weight loss without taking these supplements, but to help you feel full longer, fight cravings, and lose weight faster I recommend:

- PGX fiber, to help you feel full longer. Begin with one before each meal. Slowly work your way up to two to four capsules until desired feeling of fullness is achieved. It is best taken with 8 to 16 ounces of water, except for evening snack. Use only 8 ounces of water with your evening snack since 16 ounces may interfere with sleep.* (See Appendix B.)

- Serotonin Max or 5-HTP to help with food cravings. Take one capsule with your midafternoon snack or with your evening meal or evening snack (if craving sugars or carbs). (See Appendix B.)

- N-acetyl-tyrosine, 500 milligrams, two to three tablets thirty minutes before breakfast and thirty minutes before lunch if hunger and appetite are a problem. (See Appendix B.)

- Living Green Tea with EGCG, to help boost metabolism and possibly burn fat faster. Take one capsule three times a day. (See Appendix B.)

DR. COLBERT'S HEALTHY SALAD DRESSING

- ¼ cup organic extra-virgin olive oil
- ¾ cup balsamic vinaigrette (or other vinegar if preferred)
- Juice of ½–1 lemon or lime
- ¼ cup cilantro leaves (optional)
- 1–2 garlic cloves, pressed (or as many as desired for taste)
- Salt and pepper to taste (use Himalayan sea salt)

Mix all ingredients and transfer to a salad spritzer bottle. Makes 1 cup, which should last three months refrigerated.

---

* If you can only afford one supplement, PGX fiber is the most important one. The most critical times to take it are before your afternoon snack, evening meal, and evening snack.

Recommended protein powders and protein bars (all are optional)

I do not recommend soy-based protein. Instead, try chocolate- or vanilla-flavored whey protein powder or plant protein, which contains hemp, rice, and pea proteins; this can also be added to oatmeal or cereal. (See Appendix B.)

Kefir and fruit (blend plain low-fat kefir with fruit)

- So Delicious Coconut Milk Kefir, So Delicious Cultured Coconut Milk, Lifeway Organic kefir, low-fat plain: 8 ounces
- One medium apple or ¼ cup berries

Cheese, fruit, and nuts

- 1–2 slices of low-fat or fat-free cheese with 1 medium Granny Smith apple and 5–10 pecans, walnuts, almonds, or macadamia nuts

DR. COLBERT'S HEALTHY SMOOTHIE

If you feel you are too busy to eat breakfast, here's an easy recipe for a kefir and fruit smoothie that only takes two minutes to prepare. Combine the following ingredients in a blender for a healthy breakfast or snack:

- 8 oz. low-fat coconut kefir, cultured coconut milk, or coconut milk* (also for midmorning or midafternoon snack only; for evening snack, use 4 oz. water and 4 oz. coconut milk, cultured coconut milk, or coconut kefir)
- ¼ cup frozen blueberries, blackberries, strawberries, or raspberries (omit for evening snack)
- 1–2 Tbsp. ground flaxseeds (omit for evening snack)
- 1 scoop of chocolate- or vanilla-flavored whey protein powder or plant protein

Note: You can find more recipes like these at www.thecandodiet.com.

Make sure that the coconut milk has only 80 calories per cup.

RESOURCE GUIDE FOR REVERSING DIABETES

Most of the products mentioned throughout this book are offered through Dr. Colbert's Divine Health Wellness Center or are available at your local health food store.

Divine Health Nutritional Products
1908 Boothe Circle
Longwood, FL 32750
Phone: (407) 331-7007
Web site: www.drcolbert.com
E-mail: info@drcolbert.com

Maintenance nutritional supplements
- Divine Health Multivitamin
- Divine Health Living Multivitamin
- Max N-Fuse

Diabetic support
- PGX fiber
- Cinnulin PF (cinnamon extract)
- Divine Health Fiber
- Divine Health Nutrients for Glucose Regulation
- Divine Health Vitamin D_3, 2,000 IU
- Chromium, 200 mcg
- Alpha lipoic acid (ALA Max, 600 mg capsule)
- Diaxinol (alpha lipoic acid, cinnulin, chromium, biotin, gymnema, and vanadyl sulfate)—Dr. Colbert's favorite supplement for diabetics

Omega oils
- Divine Health Living Omega
- Ultra Krill

Recommended natural sweeteners
- Stevia
- Just Like Sugar

Protein powders
- Divine Health Undenatured Whey Protein
- Plant protein

Supplements for weight loss
- Irvingia
- PGX fiber
- Living Green Tea with EGCG

Supplements for thyroid support
- Metabolic Advantage

To curb food cravings
- Serotonin Max
- N-acetyl L-tyrosine
- Advanced fat loss drops

Other supplements
- DIM
- Indole-3-carbinol
- Beta TCP
- Divine Health Probiotic
- Divine Health Fiber Formula
- Serotonin Max
- L-carnitine with lipoic acid and PQQ (Mitochondria Basics with PQQ)

Glutathione boosters
- Max GXL
- Max One
- Cellgevity—Dr. Colbert's favorite glutathione booster

Snack bars
- Nutiva Hemp Chocolate Bars

Other Resources

- Sage Medical Lab and ALCAT for delayed food allergy/ sensitivity testing. Visit their websites at www.sagemedlab .com and www.alcat.com respectively.

- For knowledgeable doctors in bioidentical hormone replacement (make sure they are board certified in anti-aging): www.worldhealth.net

- Grissini breadsticks, which are available at most grocery stores

- hCG sublingual tablets, which must be prescribed by a physician (Physicians, call Pharmacy Specialist at (407) 260-7002.)

- Certified personal trainer. Lee Viersen is my personal trainer, and he can be reached through his website at www .LeeViersen.com or by phone at (407) 435-7059.

NOTES

Introduction—Type 2 Diabetes *Can* Be Reversed!

1. Centers for Disease Control and Prevention (CDC), "National Diabetes Fact Sheet, 2011" http://www.cdc.gov/diabetes/pubs/pdf/ndfs_2011 .pdf (accessed November 1, 2011).

2. Ibid.

3. Centers for Disease Control and Prevention (CDC), "FastStats: Obesity and Overweight," http://www.cdc.gov/nchs/fastats/overwt.htm (accessed November 1, 2011).

1—The Diabetes Epidemic

1. Wikipedia, s.v. "Super Size Me," http://en.wikipedia.org/wiki/ Supersize_me (accessed November 1, 2011).

2. Mary Clare Jalonick, "Obesity Rates Still Rising," *Huffington Post*, July 7, 2011, http://www.huffingtonpost.com/2011/07/07/obesity-states -rates_n_892181.html (accessed July 16, 2011).

3. Centers for Disease Control and Prevention (CDC), "Overweight and Obesity: U.S. Obesity Trends," http://www.cdc.gov/obesity/data/trends.html (accessed November 1, 2011).

4. A. Modad et al., "Actual Causes of Death in the United States, 2000," *Journal of the American Medical Association* 291 (2004): 1238–1245.

5. Catherine Pearson, "Smoking Rates: Pack-A-Day Smoking Is Down Dramatically," *Huffington Post,* March 16, 2011, http://www.huffingtonpost .com/2011/03/16/smoking-rates-_n_835536.html (accessed July 16, 2011).

6. Associated Press, "Obesity Rates in U.S. Leveling Off," MSNBC.com, November 28, 2007, http://www.msnbc.msn.com/id/22007477/ns/health -diet_and_nutrition/t/obesity-rates-us-leveling (accessed November 1, 2011).

7. Centers for Disease Control and Prevention (CDC), "National Diabetes Fact Sheet, 2011."

8. Ibid.

9. World Health Organization, "Diabetes Fact Sheet," http://www.who .int/mediacentre/factsheets/fs312/en/ (accessed November 1, 2011).

10. Centers for Disease Control and Prevention (CDC), "National Diabetes Fact Sheet, 2011."

11. Centers for Disease Control and Prevention (CDC), "Overweight and Obesity: Defining Overweight and Obesity," http://www.cdc.gov/obesity/defining.html (accessed November 1, 2011).

12. Gabriel I. Uwaifo, "Obesity," eMedicine.com, October 27, 2011, http://emedicine.medscape.com/article/123702-overview (accessed November 1, 2011).

13. Weight-Control Information Network, National Institute of Diabetes and Digestive and Kidney Diseases (NIDDK), "Overweight and Obesity Statistics: Economic Costs Related to Overweight and Obesity," http://win.niddk.nih.gov/statistics/#what (accessed November 1, 2011).

14. Michael S. Rosenwald, "Why America Has to Be Fat," *Washington Post,* Jan. 22, 2006, F-1.

15. Michael Pollan, *In Defense of Food: An Eater's Manifesto* (New York: Penguin Press, 2008), 116.

16. ScienceDaily.com, "Breast Cancer More Aggressive in Obese Women, Study Suggests," March 14, 2008, http://www.sciencedaily.com/releases/2008/03/080314085045.htm (accessed November 1, 2011).

17. Eric Schlosser, *Fast Food Nation* (New York: Houghton Mifflin, 2001), 3, 242.

18. Centers for Disese Control and Prevention (CDC), "Adolescent and School Health: Childhood Obesity Facts," http://www.cdc.gov/healthyyouth/obesity/facts.htm (accessed November 1, 2011).

19. K. M. Venkat Narayan, James P. Boyle, Theodore J. Thompson, Stephen W. Sorensen, and David F. Williamson, "Lifetime Risk for Diabetes Mellitus in the United States," *Journal of the American Medical Association* 290, no. 14 (2003): 1884–1890; abstract viewed at http://jama.ama-assn.org/content/290/14/1884.abstract (accessed November 1, 2011).

20. United States Department of Health and Human Services, Office of the Surgeon General, "Overweight in Children and Adolescents," http://www.surgeongeneral.gov/topics/obesity/calltoaction/fact_adolescents.htm (accessed November 1, 2011).

21. Woodruff Health Sciences Center, "Excess Fat Puts Patients with Type 2 Diabetes at Greater Risk," March 26, 2009, http://shared.web.emory.edu/whsc/news/releases/2009/03/excess-fat-puts-diabetic-patients-at-risk.html (accessed November 1, 2011).

22. ScienceDaily.com, "Obesity Increases Cancer Risk, Analysis of Hundreds of Studies Shows," February 17, 2008, http://www.sciencedaily.com/releases/2008/02/080217211802.htm (accessed November 1, 2011).

23. The Healthier Life.com, "GERD: Obesity Can Increase Your Risk of Acid Reflux Disease," March 29, 2006, http://www.thehealthierlife.co.uk/natural-health-articles/digestive-problems/gerd-obesity-increase-risk-00212.html (accessed November 1, 2011).

24. Frank Mangano, "The Obesity-Hypertension Connection: Your Weight May be Putting You at Risk," NaturalNews.com, July 27, 2009, http://www.naturalnews.com/026702_weight_blood_pressure.html (accessed November 1, 2011).

25. Michael F. Jacobson, *Liquid Candy: How Soft Drinks Are Harming Americans' Health* (Washington DC: Center for Science in the Public Interest, 2005), 8–11.

26. Rod Taylor, Carole Schmidt, and Lynn Kaladjian, "The Beanie Factor," *Brandweek*, June 16, 1997, abstract viewed at http://business.highbeam.com/137330/article-1G1-19505915/beanie-factor (accessed November 2, 2011).

27. Dan Morse, "School Cafeterias Are Enrolling as Fast-Food Franchises," *Wall Street Journal*, July 28, 1998, B2.

28. McDonalds.ca, "FAQs," http://www.mcdonalds.ca/en/aboutus/faq.aspx (accessed November 2, 2011).

29. A. J. Stunkard et al., "An Adoption Study of Human Obesity," *New England Journal of Medicine*, 314, no. 4 (1986): 193–198.

30. National Heart, Lung, and Blood Institute, National Institutes of Health, "What Causes Overweight and Obesity?" http://www.nhlbi.nih.gov/health/health-topics/topics/obe/causes.html (accessed November 2, 2011).

31. Pamela Peeke, *Fight Fat After Forty* (New York: Viking, 2000), 58.

2—Types of Diabetes

1. Tamar Levin, "Record Level of Stress Found in College Freshmen," *New York Times*, January 26, 2011, http://www.nytimes.com/2011/01/27/education/27colleges.html (accessed November 2, 2011).

2. Centers for Disease Control and Prevention (CDC), "National Diabetes Fact Sheet, 2011."

3. National Diabetes Information Clearinghouse, "Diagnosis of Diabetes," http://diabetes.niddk.nih.gov/dm/pubs/diagnosis/ (accessed November 2, 2011).

4. Centers for Disease Control and Prevention (CDC), "National Diabetes Fact Sheet, 2011."

5. American Diabetes Association, "Living With Diabetes: A1c," http://www.diabetes.org/living-with-diabetes/treatment-and-care/blood-glucose-control/a1c/ (accessed November 2, 2011).

6. Centers for Disease Control and Prevention (CDC), "National Diabetes Fact Sheet, 2011."

7. National Diabetes Information Clearinghouse, "National Diabetes Statistics, 2011," http://diabetes.niddk.nih.gov/dm/pubs/statistics/ (accessed November 2, 2011).

8. Centers for Disease Control and Prevention (CDC), "National Diabetes Fact Sheet, 2011."

9. National Diabetes Information Clearinghouse, "National Diabetes Statistics, 2011."

3—Symptoms and Long-Term Complications of Diabetes

1. American Diabetes Association, "Diabetes Basics: Symptoms," http://www.diabetes.org/diabetes-basics/symptoms/?loc=DropDownDB-symptoms (accessed November 2, 2011).

2. Ibid.

3. American Diabetes Association, "Epidemiology of Diabetes Interventions and Complications (EDIC): Design, Implementation, and Preliminary Results of a Long-Term Follow-Up of the Diabetes Control and Complications Trial Cohort," *Diabetes Care* 22, no. 1 (January 1999): 99–111, referenced in William Davis, *Wheat: The Unhealthy Whole Grain*, book excerpt "Wheat Belly," *Life Extension*, October 2011, http://www.lef.org/magazine/mag2011/oct2011_Wheat-The-Unhealthy-Whole-Grain_01.htm (accessed November 2, 2011).

4. National Diabetes Data Group and National Institutes of Health, *Diabetes in America, 2nd edition* (Bethesda, MD: National Institutes, 1995).

5. National Institute of Neurological Diseases and Stroke, "Transient Ischemic Attack Information Page," http://www.ninds.nih.gov/disorders/tia/tia.htm (accessed November 2, 2011).

6. National Eye Institute, "Facts About Diabetic Retinopathy," http://www.nei.nih.gov/health/diabetic/retinopathy.asp (accessed November 2, 2011).

7. Centers for Disease Control and Prevention (CDC), "National Diabetes Fact Sheet, 2011."

8. Ibid.

9. Ibid.

10. Ibid.

11. Ibid.

12. Ibid.

13. Ibid.

14. Ibid.

15. K. T. Khaw, N. Wareham, R. Luben, et al., "Glycated Haemoglobin, Diabetes, and Mortality in Men in Norfolk Cohort of European Prospective Investigation of Cancer and Nutrition (EPIC-Norfolk)," *British Medical Journal* 322, no. 7277 (January 6, 2001): 15–18, referenced in Davis, *Wheat: The Unhealthy Whole Grain*, book excerpt "Wheat Belly."

4—Hidden Contributor #1: Chronic Stress and Adrenal Fatigue

1. American Psychological Association, "Mind/Body Health: Did You Know?" http://www.myedhelp.com/pdf/MindBodyConnection.pdf (accessed November 2, 2011). Lyle H. Miller and Alma Dell Smith, *The Stress Solution: An Action Plan to Manage the Stress in Your Life* (New York: Pocket Books, 1993).

2. "Stress Treatments Helps Control Type 2 Diabetes," Mercola.com, January 23, 2002, http://articles.mercola.com/sites/articles/archive/2002/01/23/stress-treatments.aspx (accessed July 29, 2009).

3. Ibid.

4. Walter Bradford Cannon, *Bodily Changes in Pain, Hunger, Fear and Rage* (New York: D. Appleton and Company, 1915).

5. Essortment.com, "Stress Relief Techniques," http://www.essortment.com/stress-relief-techniques-15897.html (accessed November 2, 2011).

6. For more information on this book, see http://www.christianbook.com/Christian/Books/product?p=1142792&event=AFF&isbn=978159997913139.

5—Hidden Contributor #2: Compromised Metabolism and Insulin Resistance

1. University of Maryland Medical Center, "Omega-6 Fatty Acids," http://www.umm.edu/altmed/articles/omega-6-000317.htm (accessed November 2, 2011).

2. National Cholesterol Education Program, "ATP III Guidelines at-a -Glance Quick Desk Reference," http://www.nhlbi.nih.gov/guidelines/ cholesterol/atglance.pdf (accessed November 2, 2011).

3. HealthDay News, "Metabolic Syndrome Doubles Heart Risk, Analysis Shows," June 27, 2011, http://healthomg.com/2011/06/27/metabolic -syndrome-doubles-heart-risk-analysis-shows/ (accessed November 2, 2011).

4. Ravi Dhingra et al., "Soft Drink Consumption and Risk of Developing Cardiometabolic Risk Factors and the Metabolic Syndrome in Middle-Aged Adults in the Community," *Circulation* 116 (2007): 480–488.

5. American Diabetes Association, "Diabetes Basics: Diabetes Statistics," http://www.diabetes.org/diabetes-basics/diabetes-statistics/?utm_source =WWW&utm_medium=DropDownDB&utm_content=Statistics&utm_ campaign=CON (accessed November 3, 2011).

6. Jeffrey P. Koplan et al., "The Continuing Epidemics of Obesity and Diabetes in the United States," *Journal of the American Medical Association* 286, no. 10 (2001): 1195–1200.

7. J. P. Boyle, "Projection of Diabetes Burden Through 2050: Impact of Changing Demography and Diseases Prevalence in the U.S.," *Diabetes Care* 24, no. 11 (2001): 1936–1940.

8. Pamela L. Lutsey et al., "Dietary Intake and the Development of Metabolic Syndrome," *Circulation* 117 (2008): 754–761.

6—Hidden Contributor #3: Inflammation, Food Allergies, and Food Sensitivities

1. Wikipedia.org, s.v. "List of Wildfires: North America," http:// en.wikipedia.org/wiki/List_of_wildfires#North_America (accessed November 9, 2011).

2. Du Huaidong et al., "Glycemic Index and Glycemic Load in Relation to Food and Nutrient Intake and Metabolic Risk Factors in a Dutch Population," *American Journal of Clinical Nutrition* 87, no. 3 (2008): 655–661.

3. Giovanni Davi et al., "Platelet Activation in Obese Women: Role of Inflammation and Oxidant Stress," *Journal of the American Medical Association* 288, no. 16 (2002): 2008–2014.

4. B. B. Duncan et al., "Atherosclerosis Risk in Communities Study Investigators: Inflammation Markers Predict Increased Weight Gain in Smoking Quitters," *Obesity Research* 11, no. 11 (November 2003): 1339–1344; and E. Barinas-Mitchell et al., "Serum Levels of C-Reactive Protein Are Associated With Obesity, Weight Gain, and Hormone Replacement Therapy in Healthy Postmenopausal Women," *American Journal of Epidemiology* 153, no. 11 (June 2001): 1094–1101.

5. G. Engstrom et al., "Inflammation-Sensitive Plasma Proteins Are Associated With Future Weight Gain," *Diabetes* 52, no. 8 (August 2003): 2097–2101.

6. Clara Felix, *All About Omega-3 Oils* (Garden City, NY: Avery Publishing, 1998), 32.

7. Simon Liu et al., "Increased Consumption of Refined Carbohydrates and the Epidemic of Type 2 Diabetes in the United States: An Ecological Assessment," *American Journal of Clinical Nutrition* 79, no. 5 (2004): 774–779.

8. Ibid.

9. Marian Burros, "Stores Say Wild Salmon, but Tests Say Farm Bred," *New York Times*, April 10, 2005, http://www.nytimes.com/2005/04/10/dining/10salmon.html?scp=1&sq=stores+say+wild+salmon&st=nyt (accessed November 9, 2011).

10. Andrea Markowitz, "Forbidden Fruits and Other Foods," *Chicago Tribune*, July 26, 2010, http://articles.chicagotribune.com/2010-07-26/health/sc-health-0723-allergies-food-20100723_1_food-intolerance-food-allergies-anaphylactic-reaction (accessed November 9, 2011).

7—Hidden Contributor #4: Hormone Imbalance

1. LifeExtension.org, "Female Hormone Restoration," January 20, 2006, http://search.lef.org/LEFCMS/aspx/PrintVersionMagic.aspx?CmsID=113516 (accessed November 3, 2011).

2. A. D. Seftel, "Male Hypogonadism, Part 1: Epidemiology of Hypogonadism," *International Journal of Impotence Research* 18, no. 2 (2006): 115–120.

3. Thomas Mulligan, "Prevalence of Hypogonadism in Males Aged at Least 45 Years: The HIM Study," *International Journal of Clinical Practice* 60 (2006): 762–769.

4. Ibid.

5. T. G. Travison et al., "The Relative Contributions of Aging, Health, and Lifestyle Factors to Serum Testosterone Decline in Men," *Journal of Clinical Endocrinology and Metabolism* (Dec. 5, 2006), referenced in Jane Collingwood, "Emotions and Weight Affect Testosterone Levels," January 8, 2007, http://psychcentral.com/lib/2007/emotions-and-weight-affect -testosterone-levels/ (accessed November 3, 2009).

6. ScienceDaily.com, "Older Men May Not Live as Long If They Have Low Testosterone," June 5, 2007, http://www.sciencedaily.com/ releases/2007/06/070605132125.htm (accessed November 3, 2011).

7. Hau Liu et al., "Systematic Review: The Effects of Growth Hormone on Athletic Performance," *Annals of Internal Medicine* 148, no. 10 (2008).

8. Daniel Rudman et al., "Effects of Human Growth Hormone in Men Over 60 Years Old," *New England Journal of Medicine* 323 (1990): 1–6.

9. Ronald Klatz with Carol Kahn, *Grow Young With HGH* (HarperCollins: New York, 1997), 5.

8—How Metabolism Works

1. "Time Lapse Photography: Interview With John Novotny," *The Campsite* (blog), April 17, 2011, http://thecampsiteblog.com/2011/04/17/time -lapse-photography/ (accessed November 3, 2011).

2. Barbara Bushman and Janice Clark-Young, *Action Plan for Menopause* (Champaign, IL: American College of Sports Medicine, 2005), 68–70.

3. Ibid.

4. *Webster's New World College Dictionary*, 4th ed. (n.p.: Wiley Publishing, Inc., 2004), s.v. "metabolism."

5. Jim Harvey, "Measuring BMR in the Pulmonary Lab," *FOCUS: Journal for Respiratory Care and Sleep Medicine* (July 1, 2006), http://www.thefreelibrary.com/Measuring+BMR+in+the+Pulmonary+ lab.-a0186218061 (accessed November 3, 2011).

6. Uwaifo, "Obesity."

7. James Levine et al., "Interindividual Variation in Posture Allocation: Possible Role in Human Obesity, *Science* 307, no. 5709 (2005): 584–586.

8. Lawrence C. Wood et al., *Your Thyroid: A Home Reference* (New York: Ballentine Books, 1995).

9. Karilee Halo Shames et al., "The Thyroid Dance: Nursing Approaches to Autoimmune Low Thyroid," *AWHONN Lifelines* 6, no 1 (2002): 52–59.

9—The Glycemic Index and Glycemic Load

1. MrBreakfast.com, "The Early Days of Breakfast Cereal," http://www.mrbreakfast.com/article.asp?articleid=13 (accessed November 3, 2011).

2. BestDietTips.com, "Glycemic Index List of Foods," http://www.bestdiettips.com/glycemic-index-food-list-high-and-low-gi-index-foods-chart (accessed November 3, 2011).

10—What About Bread and Other Carbs?

1. David Zinczenko with Matt Goulding, *Eat This, Not That!* (New York: Rodale Books, 2008), 12.

2. Matt Goulding, "The 20 Worst Foods in America: 2. Worst Starter, Chili's Awesome Blossom," http://www.menshealth.com/20worst/worststarter.html (accessed November 4, 2011).

3. U.S. Department of Health and Human Services, *Dietary Guidelines for Americans, 2005,* 6th ed., (Washington, DC: U.S. Government Printing Office, 2005).

4. Neal Bernard, *Breaking the Food Seduction* (New York: St. Martin's Press, 2003), 32.

5. John Casey, WebMD Weight Loss Clinic, "The Hidden Ingredient That Can Sabotage Your Diet," http://www.medicinenet.com/script/main/art.asp?articlekey=56589 (accessed November 4, 2011).

6. Becky Hand, "The Hunt for Hidden Sugar," BabyFit.com, http://babyfit.sparkpeople.com/articles.asp?id=685 (accessed November 4, 2011).

7. My Fox NY, "Teens' Sugar Intake Poses Health Risks," January 12, 2011, http://www.myfoxny.com/dpps/news/teens-sugar-intake-raises-health-risks-dpgonc-20110112-gc_11410193 (accessed November 4, 2011).

8. Gary Taubes, "Is Sugar Toxic?" *New York Times Magazine*, April 13, 2011, http://www.nytimes.com/2011/04/17/magazine/mag-17Sugar-t.html? (accessed November 4, 2011).

9. Sucralose.org, "Your Questions Answered," http://www.sucralose.org/questions/ (accessed November 4, 2011).

10. Sally Fallon Morell and Rami Nagel, "Worse Than We Thought: The Lowdown on High-Fructose Corn Syrup and Agave Nectar," *Wise Traditions*, Spring 2009, 44–51, http://allnaturalpediatrics.com/Documents/HFCS%20article.pdf (accessed November 4, 2011).

11—What You Need to Know About Fiber and Fats

1. James W. Anderson, *Dr. Anderson's High-Fiber Fitness Plan* (Lexington, KY: University Press of Kentucky, 1994), 14.

2. Institute of Medicine, *Dietary Reference Intakes for Energy, Carbohydrate, Fiber, Fat, Fatty Acids, Cholesterol, Protein, and Amino Acids* (Washington DC: The National Academies Press, 2002).

3. Nancy C. Howarth et al., "Dietary Fat and Fiber Are Associated With Excess Weight in Young and Middle-Aged U.S. Adults," *Journal of the American Dietetic Association* 105, no. 9 (2005): 1365–1372.

4. USDA Center for Nutrition Policy and Promotion, "Is Total Fat Consumption Really Decreasing?" *Nutrition Insights* 5 (April 1998), http://www.cnpp.usda.gov/Publications/NutritionInsights/insight5.pdf (accessed November 4, 2011).

5. Crisco.com, "Our History," http://www.crisco.com/About_Crisco/History.aspx (accessed November 4, 2011).

6. Associated Press, "Crisco Drops Trans Fat From Shortening Formula," MSNBC.com, January 25, 2007, http://www.msnbc.msn.com/id/16795455/ns/health-diet_and_nutrition/t/crisco-drops-trans-fats-shortening-formula/ (accessed November 4, 2011).

7. Jane E. Brody, "Women's Heart Risk Linked to Types of Fats, Not Total," *New York Times*, November 20, 1997, http://www.nytimes.com/specials/women/warchive/971120_1599.html (accessed November 4, 2011).

8. Wendy DeMark-Wahnefried, ABC News, "A Donut for Your Diet? The Truth About Trans Fat," August 28, 2007, http://abcnews.go.com/Health/Diet/story?id=3121351&page=1 (accessed November 4, 2011).

9. Electronic Code of Federal Regulations, "Title 21: Food and Drugs, Section 101.9 Nutrition Labeling of Food," http://www.accessdata.fda.gov/scripts/cdrh/cfdocs/cfCFR/CFRSearch.cfm?fr=101.9 (accessed November 4, 2011).

10. American Heart Association, "Step I Diet: TLC Guidelines," http://www.livestrong.com/article/390572-step-i-diet/ (accessed November 4, 2011).

11. Anthony Kane, "Omega-3 Fatty Acids and Depression," ADDADHDAdvances.com, http://addadhdadvances.com/efa-depression.html (accessed November 7, 2011).

12. Ancel Keys, *Seven Countries: A Multivariate Analysis of Death and Coronary Heart Disease* (Boston: Harvard University Press, 1980).

13. Tinker Ready, "Dueling Diets," *Harvard Public Health Review* (Fall 2004); Elizabeth Somer, "Pass the Olive Oil," Apr. 30, 2001, http://www.greekfamilyoil.weebly.com/should-i-consume-olive-oil-if-im-trying-to-lose-weight.html (accessed November 7, 2011).

12—Beverages: Are You Drinking Your Way to Diabetes?

1. American Beverage Association, "What America Drinks," http://improveyourhealthwithwater.info/a1/whatamericadrinks.pdf (accessed November 7, 2011).

2. Ibid.

3. Judith Valentine, "Soft Drinks: America's Other Drinking Problem," DetoxifyNow.com, http://www.detoxifynow.com/soft_drink_dangers.html (accessed November 7, 2011).

4. Daniel J. DeNoon, "Drink More Diet Soda, Gain More Weight?" WebMD.com, June 13, 2005, http://www.webmd.com/diet/news/20050613/drink-more-diet-soda-gain-more-weight (accessed November 7, 2011).

5. Lutsey et al., "Dietary Intake and the Development of Metabolic Syndrome."

6. Jacobson, *Liquid Candy: How Soft Drinks Are Harming Americans' Health.*

7. Ibid.

8. Centers for Disease Control and Prevention (CDC), "Overweight and Obesity, Data and Statistics," http://www.cdc.gov/obesity/childhood/data.html (accessed November 7, 2011).

9. R. Dhingra et al., "Soft Drink Consumption and Risk of Developing Cardiometabolic Risk Factors and the Metabolic Syndrome in Middle-Aged Adults in the Community," *Circulation* 116, no. 5 (July 2007): 480–488.

10. Jacobson, *Liquid Candy: How Soft Drinks Are Harming Americans' Health.*

11. Zinczenko, *Eat This, Not That!* 258.

12. Starbucks.com, "Explore Our Menu," http://www.starbucks.com/menu/catalog/nutrition?drink=all#view_control=nutriton (accessed November 7, 2011).

13. R. M. van Dam and E. J. M. Feskens, "Coffee Consumption and Risk of Type 2 Diabetes Mellitus," *Lancet* 360, no. 9344 (November 2002): 1477–1478, referenced in Dave Tuttle, "Controlling Blood Sugar With Cinnamon and Coffee Berry," *Life Extension*, December 2005, http://www.lef.org/magazine/mag2005/dec2005_report_cinnamon_01.htm (accessed November 7, 2011).

14. J. Tuomilchto, G. Hu, S. Bidel, J. Lindstrom, and P. Jousilahti, "Coffee Consumption and Risk of Type 2 Diabetes Mellitus Among Middle-Aged Finnish Men and Women," *Journal of the American Medical Association* 291, no. 10 (March 2004): 1213–1219, referenced in Tuttle, "Controlling Blood Sugar With Cinnamon and Coffee Berry."

15. Y. Kobayashi et al., "Green Tea Polyphenols Inhibit the Sodium-Dependent Glucose Transporter of Intestinal Epithelial Cells by a Competitive Mechanism," *Journal of Agricultural and Food Chemistry* 48, no. 11 (November 2000): 5618–5623, referenced in Tuttle, "Controlling Blood Sugar With Cinnamon and Coffee Berry."

16. Mayo Clinic Staff, "Caffeine: How Much Is Too Much?", MayoClinic.com, http://www.mayoclinic.com/health/caffeine/NU00600 (accessed November 7, 2011).

17. John Tesh, *Intelligence for Your Life* (Nashville: Thomas Nelson Publishers, 2008), 121.

18. MyFitnessPal.com, "Calories in Gatorade g Series Pro 01 Prime Carb Energy Drink Fruit Punch," http://www.myfitnesspal.com/food/calories/gatorade-g-series-pro-01-prime-carb-energy-drink-fruit-punch-3719780 (accessed November 7, 2011).

19. Health4YouOnline.com, "Dehydration—the Benefits of Drinking Water," http://www.health4youonline.com/article_dehydration.htm (accessed November 7, 2011).

20. Susanna C. Larsson and Alicja Wolk, "Tea Consumption and Ovarian Cancer Risk in a Population-Based Cohort," *Archives of Internal Medicine* 165, no. 22 (December 12, 2005): 2683–2686, http://archinte.ama-assn.org/cgi/reprint/165/22/2683.pdf (accessed November 7, 2011).

21. Abdul G. Dulloo et al., "Efficacy of a Green Tea Extract Rich in Catechin Polyphenols and Caffeine in Increasing 24-h Energy Expenditure and Fat Oxidation in Humans," *American Journal of Clinical Nutrition* 70, no. 6 (December 1999): 1040–1045.

22. Jukka Hintakka et al., "Daily Tea Drinking Is Associated With a Low Level of Depressive Symptoms in the Finnish General Population," *European Journal of Epidemiology* 20, no. 4 (2005): 359–363.

23. Guayaki.com, "All About Mate: Health Benefits," http://guayaki.com/mate/2931/Health-Benefits.html (accessed November 7, 2011).

13—Your Waist and Your Weight: Powerful Keys to Reversing Diabetes

1. Linda K. "Tallest, Fastest, Longest: Top 10 Roller Coasters in America," *Uptake* (blog), http://attractions.uptake.com/blog/top-10-roller -coasters-4014.html (accessed November 7, 2011).

2. Lauren Muney, "Top 10 Excuses for Falling off the Diet/Fitness Wagon—and Answer for Them," PhysicalMind.com, http://www .physicalmind.com/articles.html (accessed November 7, 2011).

3. Centers for Disease Control and Prevention (CDC), "Overweight and Obesity: Defining Overweight and Obesity."

4. Youfa Wang et al., "Comparison of Abdominal Adiposty and Overall Obesity in Predicting Risk of Type 2 Diabetes Among Men," *American Journal of Clinical Nutrition* 81, No. 3 (2005): 555–563.

14—Catch the Vision for the New You

1. Amanda Spake, "The Belly Burden," *U.S. News & World Report*, November 20, 2005, http://health.usnews.com/usnews/health/articles/051128/28waist.htm (accessed November 7, 2011).

2. Krisha McCoy, "Your Body Fat Percentage: What Does It Mean?" HealthLibrary.com, January 18, 2011, http://healthlibrary.epnet.com/GetContent.aspx?token=1edc3d6e-4fec-4b20-baca-795e48830daa&chunkiid =41373 (accessed November 7, 2011).

17—Rapid Waist Reduction Diet, Phase Two

1. American College of Obstetricians and Gynecologists, "Nutrition During Pregnancy," patient education information sheet, June 2008.

2. Lynn R. Goldman et al., "American Academy of Pediatrics: Technical Report: Mercury in the Environment: Implications for Pediatricians," *Pediatrics* 108, no. 1 (July 2001): 197–205.

18—Treats and Cheats

1. Jennie Brand-Miller, Thomas M. S. Wolever, Kay Foster-Powell, and Stephen Colagiuri, *The New Glucose Revolution*, 3rd ed., (New York: Marlow & Co., 2007), 86.

2. Charles Stuart Platkin, *The Automatic Diet* (New York: Hudson Street Press, 2005), 92.

3. Maria Conceicao de Oliveira et al., "Weight Loss Association With a Daily Intake of Three Apples or Three Pears Among Overweight Women," *Nutrition* 19, no. 3 (2003): 253–256.

4. Judith J. Wurtman and Nina Frusztajer Marquis, *The Serotonin Power Diet* (New York: Rodale, 2006), 15.

5. Ibid., 66–68.

19—Tips for Eating Out and Grocery Shopping

1. National Restaurant Association, "Restaurant Industry Sales Turn Positive in 2011 After Three Tough Years," PRNewswire, February 1, 2011, http://multivu.prnewswire.com/mnr/national-restaurant-association/42965/ (accessed November 8, 2011).

2. National Restaurant Association, "National Restaurant Association's First-of-Its-Kind "Kids LiveWell" Initiative Showcases Restaurants' Healthful Menu Options for Children," press release, July 13, 2011, http://www .restaurant.org/pressroom/pressrelease/?ID=2136 (accessed November 8, 2011).

3. Rich Pirog, Timothy Van Pelt, Kamyar Enshayan, and Ellen Cook, "Food, Fuel, and Freeways: An Iowa Perspective on How Far Food Travels, Fuel Usage, and Greenhouse Gas Emissions," Leopold Center for Sustainable Agriculture, June 2001, http://www.leopold.iastate.edu/pubs-and-papers/2001-06-food-fuel-freeways (accessed November 9, 2011).

4. Tanya Zuckerbrot, "Did You Know? Frozen Can Be Healthier Than Fresh," FOXNews.com, December 14, 2011, http://www.foxnews.com/ health/2011/12/14/did-know-frozen-can-be-healthier-than-fresh/ (accessed December 19, 2011).

5. Paul Kita, "The Sad State of the Frozen Meal, Part 1," *Guy Gourmet* (blog), March 9, 2010, http://blogs.menshealth.com/guy-gourmet/gut -check-the-sad-state-of-the-frozen-meal-part-i/2010/03/09/ (accessed November 9, 2011).

6. SupermarketGuru.com, "The Things You Need to Know About Frozen Dinners," April 4, 2007, http://archive.supermarketguru.com/page .cfm/32858 (accessed November 9, 2011).

20—Supplements to Reverse Diabetes

1. Madison Park, "Half of Americans Use Supplements," CNN.com, April 13, 2011, http://www.cnn.com/2011/HEALTH/04/13/supplements .dietary/index.html (accessed November 9, 2011).

2. ScienceDaily.com, "Vitamin D Is the 'It' Nutrient of the Moment," January 12, 2009, http://www.sciencedaily.com/ releases/2009/01/090112121821.htm (accessed November 9, 2011).

3. Office of Dietary Supplements, "Dietary Supplement Fact Sheet: Chromium," http://ods.od.nih.gov/factsheets/chromium (accessed November 9, 2011).

4. Neal D. Barnard, *Dr. Neal Barnard's Program for Reversing Diabetes* (New York: Rodale, 2007), 142.

5. Office of Dietary Supplements, "Dietary Supplement Fact Sheet: Chromium."

6. Richard Anderson, Noella Bryden, and Marilyn Polansky, "Stability and Absorption of Chromium and Absorption of Chromium Histidine by Humans," *Biological Trace Elements Research* 101 (August 1, 2004): 211–218.

7. Barnard, *Dr. Neal Barnard's Program for Reversing Diabetes*, 143.

8. Richard A. Anderson, "Chromium in the Prevention and Control of Diabetes," *Diabetes and Metabolism* 26, no. 1 (February 2000): 22–27.

9. Ibid.

10. Richard A. Anderson, "Chromium, Glucose Intolerance and Diabetes," *Journal of the American College of Nutrition* 17, no. 6 (1998): 548–555, http://www.jacn.org/content/17/6/548.full (accessed November 9, 2011).

11. Mark A. Mitchell, "Lipoic Acid: A Multitude of Metabolic Health Benefits," *Life Extension*, October 2007, http://www.lef.org/magazine/ mag2007/oct2007_nu_lipoic_acid_01.htm (accessed November 9, 2011).

12. A. Khan et al., "Cinnamon Improves Glucose and Lipids in People With Type 2 Diabetes," *Diabetes Care* 26 (2003): 3215–3218, referenced in John R. White, "Cinnamon: Should It Be Taken as a Diabetes Medication?" *Diabetes Health*, December 25, 2008, http://www.diabeteshealth.com/

read/2008/12/25/5703/cinnamon-should-it-be-taken-as-a-diabetes
-medication/ (accessed November 9, 2011).

13. Mike Adams, "Study Shows Cinnulin Promotes Increase in Lean
Body Mass and Reduction in Body Fat," NaturalNews.com, September
26, 2005, http://www.naturalnews.com/011852.html (accessed November 9,
2011).

14. U. Riserus, W. C. Willett, and F. B. Hu, "Dietary Fats and Prevention
of Type 2 Diabetes," *Progress in Lipid Research* 48, no. 1 (January 2009):
44–51.

15. Dale Kiefer, "Benfotiamine," *Life Extension*, January 2007, http://
www.lef.org/magazine/mag2007/jan2007_report_benfotiamine_01.htm
(accessed November 9, 2011).

21—Supplements That Support Weight Loss

1. Michael Johnson, "Obesity Epidemic Feeds Weight-Loss Product
Sales," DrugStoreNews.com, January 5, 2011, http://www.drugstorenews
.com/article/obesity-epidemic-feeds-weight-loss-product-sales (accessed
November 9, 2011).

2. Stephen Bent, Thomas N. Tiedt, Michelle C. Odden, and Michael G.
Shlipak, "The Relative Safety of Ephedra Compared With Other Herbal
Products," *Annals of Internal Medicine* 138, no. 6 (March 18, 2003): 468–
471, http://www.annals.org/content/138/6/468.full (accessed November 9,
2011).

3. Associated Press, "FDA Warns Consumers to Avoid Brazilian Diet
Pills," USAToday.com, January 13, 2006, http://www.usatoday.com/news/
health/2006-01-13-brazilian-diet-pills_x.htm (accessed November 9, 2011).

4. Ano Lobb, "Hepatoxicity Associated With Weight-Loss Supplements:
A Case for Better Post-Marketing Surveillance, *World Journal of
Gastroenterology* 15, no. 14 (April 14, 2009): 1786–1787, http://www.ncbi
.nlm.nih.gov/pmc/articles/PMC2668789/ (accessed November 9, 2011).

5. Julius Goepp, "Critical Need for a Multi-Modal Approach to Combat
Obesity," *Life Extension*, June 2009, http://www.lef.org/magazine/
mag2009/jun2009_Multi-Modal-Approach-To-Combat-Obesity_01.htm
(accessed November 9, 2011).

6. P. Chantre and D. Lairon, "Recent Findings of Green Tea
Extract AR25 (Exolise) and Its Activity for the Treatment of Obesity,"
Phytomedicine 9, no. 1 (2002): 3–8.

7. Goepp, "Critical Need For a Multi-Modal Approach to Combat Obesity."

8. Z. Ramazanov, "Effect of Fucoxanthin and Xanthigen, A Phytomedicine Containing Fucoxanthin and Pomegranate Seed Oil, on Energy Expenditure in Obese Non-Diabetic Female Volunteers: A Double-Blind, Randomized and Placebo-Controlled Trial." Submitted for publication 2008.

9. Ibid.

10. American Thyroid Association, "Iodine Deficiency," http://www .thyroid.org/patients/patient_brochures/iodine_deficiency.html (accessed November 9, 2011).

11. Lisa Bolton et al., "How Does Drug and Supplement Marketing Affect a Healthy Lifestyle?" *Journal of Consumer Research* 34 (2008).

12. Judith A. Marlett et al., "Position of the American Dietetic Association: Health Implications of Dietary Fiber," *Journal of the American Dietetic Association* 102, no. 7 (2002): 993–1000.

13. N. C. Howarth et al., "Dietary Fiber and Weight Regulation," *Nutrition Review* 59, no. 5 (2001): 129–138.

14. Life Extension, "Obesity: Strategies to Fight a Rising Epidemic," http://www.lef.org/protocols/metabolic_health/obesity_01.htm (accessed November 9, 2011).

15. Judith N. Ngondi et al., "IGOB131, a Novel Seed Extract of the West African Plant Irvingia Gabonensis, Significantly Reduces Body Weight and Improves Metabolic Parameters in Overweight Humans in a Randomized Double-Blind Placebo Controlled Investigation," *Lipids in Health and Disease* 8, no. 7 (March 2009): http://www.lipidworld.com/content/8/1/7 (accessed November 9, 2011).

16. Hoodia Advice, "The Science of Hoodia," http://www.hoodia-advice .org/hoodia-plant.html (accessed November 9, 2011).

17. Tom Mangold, "Sampling the Kalahari Hoodia Diet," BBC News, May 30, 2003, http://news.bbc.co.uk/2/hi/programmes/ correspondent/2947810.stm (accessed November 9, 2011).

22—The Importance of Activity

1. TMZ.com, "Janet in Shape and in 'Control,'" July 27, 2006, http:// www.tmz.com/2006/07/17/janet-in-shape-and-in-control/ (accessed March 15, 2008).

2. Rob Carnevale, "Bruce Willis: Die Hard 4.0," BBC, July 2, 2007, http://www.bbc.co.uk/films/2007/07/02/bruce_willis_die_hard_4_2007_interview.shtml (accessed November 9, 2011).

3. Starpulse.com, "Memorable Celebrity Quotes," January 16, 2008, http://www.starpulse.com/news/index.php/2008/01/16/memorable_celebrity_quotes_118 (accessed November 9, 2011).

4. Mirelle Agaman, "Exclusive: Serena Williams Talks to Star!," *Star*, May 4, 2007, http://www.starmagazine.com/news/exclusive-serena-williams-talks-star (accessed November 9, 2011).

5. Stephen Miller, "Jack LaLanne, Media Fitness Guru, Dies at 96," *Wall Street Journal*, January 24, 2011, http://online.wsj.com/article/SB1000142405274870339850457610092313505768.html (accessed November 9, 2011).

6. Centers for Disease Control and Prevention (CDC), "U.S. Physical Activity Statistics," http://apps.nccd.cdc.gov/PASurveillance/StateSumV.asp (accessed November 9, 2011).

7. Jacqueline Stenson, "Excuses, Excuses," MSNBC.com, December 16, 2004, http://www.msnbc.msn.com/id/6391079/ns/health-fitness/t/excuses-excuses/ (accessed November 9, 2011); Chad Clark, "Functional Exercise: Top 10 List of Reasons Why People Don't Exercise," http://pt-connections.com/topfit/publish/printer_functional_exercise_top_10_reasons.shtml (accessed November 9, 2011).

8. Centers for Disease Control and Prevention (CDC), "Physical Activity for Everyone," http://www.cdc.gov/physicalactivity/everyone/guidelines/adults.html (accessed November 9, 2011).

9. Jennifer Corbett Dooren, "New Exercise Goal: 60 Minutes a Day," *Wall Street Journal*, March 24, 2010, http://online.wsj.com/article/SB100014240527487048961045751400111148266470.html (accessed November 9, 2011).

10. Zinczenko, *Eat This, Not That!* 113.

11. Ming Wei et al., "The Association Between Cardiorespiratory Fitness and Impaired Fasting Glucose and Type 2 Diabetes Mellitus in Men," *Annals of Internal Medicine* 130, no. 2 (January 19, 1999): 89–96, http://www.annals.org/content/130/2/89.abstract (accessed November 9, 2011).

12. Lindsay Bergstrom, "70-year-old Swims English Channel to Promote Church's Ministry in Haiti," Associated Baptist Press, September 1, 2004, http://www.abpnews.com/index.php?option=com_content&task=view&id=1863&Itemid=117 (accessed November 9, 2011).

13. Levine, "Interindividual Variation in Posture Allocation: Possible Role in Human Obesity."

14. MedicalNewsToday.com, "Blood Sugar Lowered by Brief, High-Intensity Workouts in Diabetics," December 14, 2011, http://www.medicalnewstoday.com/releases/239101.php (accessed December 19, 2011).

15. Cris A. Slentz et al., "Effects of the Amount of Exercise on Body Weight, Body Composition, and Measures of Central Obesity," *Archives of Internal Medicine* 164 (2004): 31–39.

16. Caroline J. Cedarquist, "Fitness With Fido: A Healthy Pastime for Dog Owners," NewsBlaze.com, January 10, 2006, http://newsblaze.com/story/20060110091932nnnn.nb/topstory.html (accessed November 9, 2011).

17. L. E. Davidson et al., "Effects of Exercise Modality on Insulin Resistance and Functional Limitation in Older Adults," *Archives of Internal Medicine* 169, no. 2 (January 26, 2009): 122–131, http://archinte.ama-assn.org/cgi/content/full/169/2/122 (accessed November 9, 2011).

18. Berit L. Heitmann and Peter Frederiksen, "Thigh Circumference and Risk of Heart Disease and Premature Death: Prospective Cohort Study," *British Medical Journal* 339 (September 3, 2009): http://www.bmj.com/content/339/bmj.b3292 (accessed November 9, 2011).

19. K. Boutelle and D. Kirschenbaum, "Further Support for Consistent Self-Monitoring as a Vital Component of Successful Weight Control," *Obesity Research* 6, no. 3 (May 1998): 219–224, http://www.ncbi.nlm.nih.gov/pubmed/9618126 (accessed November 9, 2011).

INDEX

Symbols

5-hydroxytryptophan (5-HTP) 175, 206

A

ACE inhibitor 27

acid reflux (GERD) 12, 34, 62

Addison's disease 37

adrenal fatigue 32-40

adrenaline 34-35

advanced glycation end-products (AGEs) 28-29, 198

Alzheimer's disease 10, 50-51, 54, 85, 117

American Diabetes Association 44, 92

American Heart Association 207

amphetamines 201, 203

amputation(s) 3, 27-28, 44

Anderson, Richard A. 196

andropause (male menopause) 70

anti-inflammatory diet 58, 160-161, 169, 210

arteriosclerosis 24

arthritis 10, 14, 50, 54, 57, 62, 214

atherosclerosis 24-25, 29, 50, 106, 198

B

basal metabolic rate (BMR) 76-78

bioidentical hormones 66, 68

bioimpedance analysis 136

birth control pills 67, 80, 145

birth defect(s) 10, 28

body fat percentage 9, 79, 134-138, 220

body mass index (BMI) 7-9, 130, 134, 136

C

caffeine 36, 116-118, 202, 204

Calorie Control Council 171

cancer(s) 8, 10, 12, 14, 30, 32, 50-51, 53-54, 63, 66-67, 72, 85, 101, 104, 120-121, 136, 145, 147, 185-186, 214

Cannizzaro, Joseph 17

Cannon, Walter 34

carpal tunnel syndrome 27, 72

Centers for Disease Control and Prevention (CDC) 1, 7-8, 11, 45, 115, 130, 213

childhood obesity 11

chronic inflammation 25, 49-51, 56, 63

chronic stress 32-40, 43, 78, 81, 175

claudication 25

cortisol 2, 33-38, 43, 51, 78-79, 175, 215, 219

C-reactive protein (CRP) 50-52, 54, 56, 58, 209-210

D

DHEA 35, 37, 72

diabetic neuropathy 24, 27, 197, 199

diabetic retinopathy 24, 26

dialysis 3, 26, 29

dopamine 207

Duke University 220

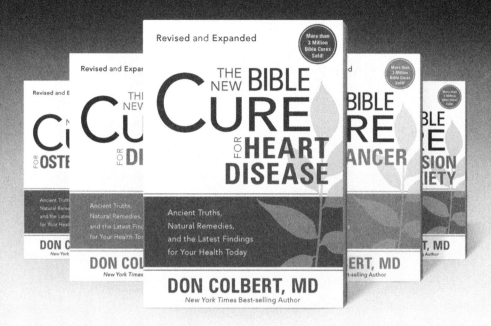

YOU WANT TO BE HEALTHY. GOD WANTS YOU TO BE HEALTHY.

In each book of the Bible Cure series, you will find helpful alternative medical information together with uplifting and faith-building biblical truths.

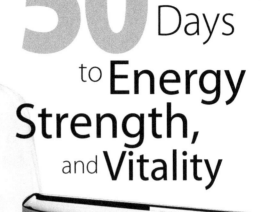
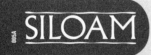